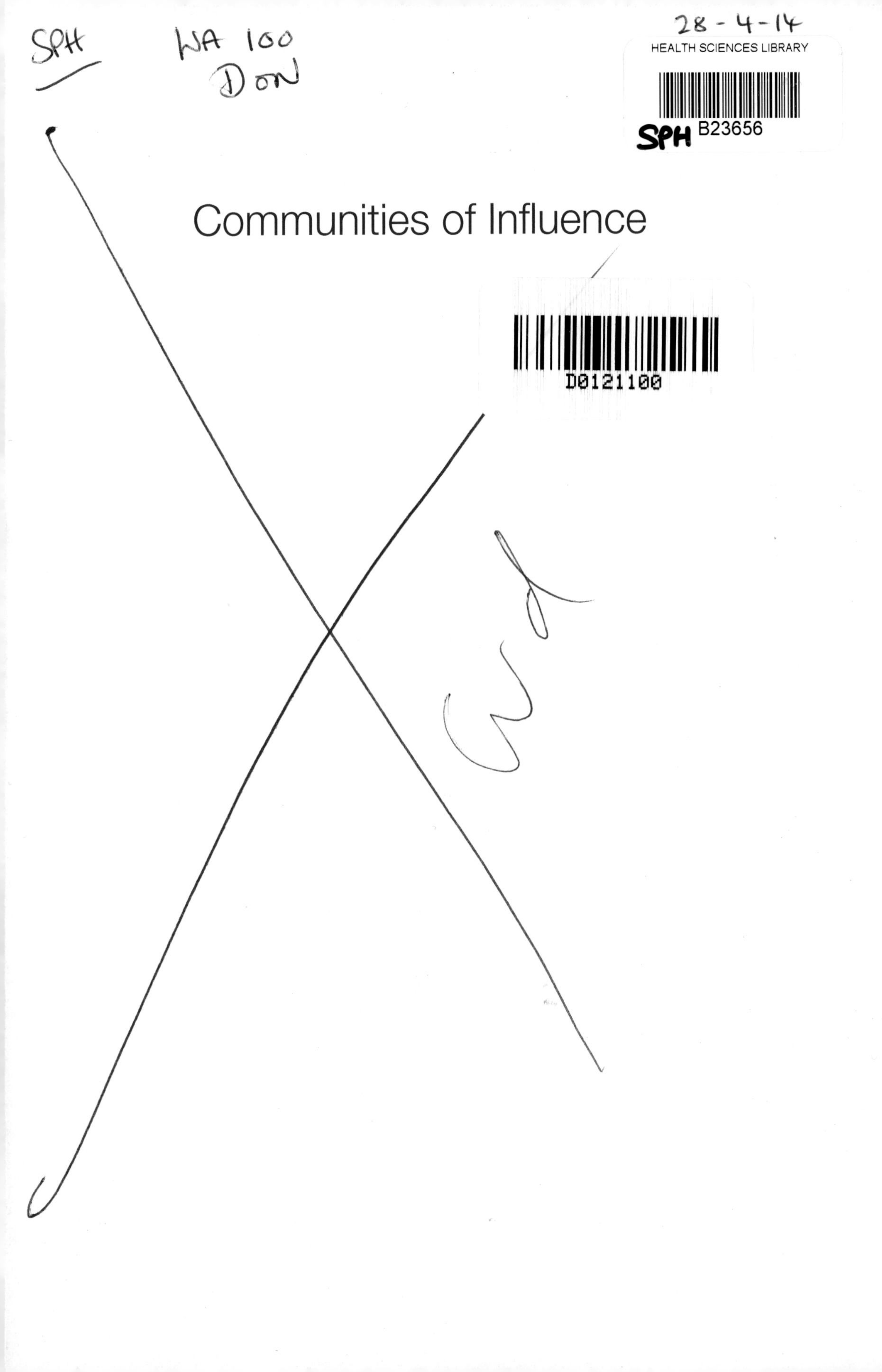



# Communities of Influence

# Communities of Influence

## IMPROVING HEALTHCARE THROUGH CONVERSATIONS AND CONNECTIONS

**ALISON DONALDSON**
*Independent expert in reflective and narrative writing*
*Visiting Research Fellow, Business School, University of Hertfordshire*

**ELIZABETH LANK**
*Independent expert in collaborative working*

*and*

**JANE MAHER**
*Consultant Clinical Oncologist*
*Chief Medical Officer, Macmillan Cancer Support*

*Foreword by*
**SIR MUIR GRAY**
*Director*
*The Oxford Centre for Healthcare Transformation*

Radcliffe Publishing
London • New York

**Radcliffe Publishing Ltd**
33–41 Dallington Street
London
EC1V 0BB
United Kingdom

**www.radcliffepublishing.com**
Electronic catalogue and worldwide online ordering facility.



British Library Cataloguing in Publication Data

A catalogue record for this book is available from the British Library.

ISBN-13: 978 184619 492 4

The paper used for the text pages of this book is FSC® certified. FSC (The Forest Stewardship Council®) is an international network to promote responsible management of the world's forests.

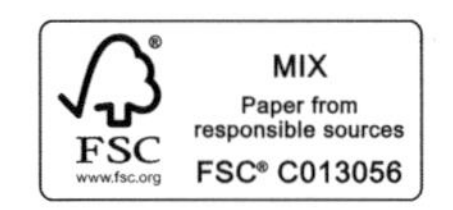


Typeset by Pindar NZ, Auckland, New Zealand
Printed and bound by TJI Digital, Padstow, Cornwall, UK

# Contents

# Foreword

For 50 years, health services have relied on two types of organisation to deliver healthcare: markets and bureaucracies. Over the years, both in the UK and in many developed countries (with the exception of the United States), the latter model has been dominant, but even the operation of the market pits bureaucracy against bureaucracy.

The rise of the bureaucracy was, to some degree, a consequence of the rise of the hospitals, the secular cathedrals of the 20th century. Big structures need a bureaucracy, and it is important to recognise the many benefits that a bureaucracy brings, provided that it adheres to the tasks for which a bureaucracy was designed, such as the open employment and promotion of staff, or the management of finance without corruption. It is when bureaucracies attempt tasks such as improving care for people with epilepsy or ensuring that people have a good death that they become ineffective, at best, or counter-productive.

There is, however, a third approach, popularised by a flurry of books and articles on complex adaptive systems published over the last few years, popularised by the ant colony. An ant colony consists of many individuals working together to solve problems for the good of the group, with individuals and groups not only behaving altruistically, but also learning to do it even better. This wonderful book describes how a creative, problem-solving organisation can be encouraged to start, grow and flourish. The authors have coined the term 'community of influence' to describe this way of working. Furthermore, it is not simply a theory; it is based on evidence from experience, which the authors have described with objectivity and appropriate detachment.

The result is a text that could act as a guide for 21st-century healthcare, one of the key books for an era in which it will be recognised that new solutions are needed for the problems we face. These solutions will not be created by bureaucracies or markets but will emerge from people working together, patients and professionals from different organisations. Communities of influence produce solutions, and this book describes how to develop them.

**Sir Muir Gray**
**Director**
**The Oxford Centre for Healthcare Transformation**
*April 2011*

# About the authors

**Alison Donaldson** has worked for the past 20 years as an independent coach and writer with a special interest in intelligent uses of writing. She started her working life in research roles in London and Berlin, then worked on *Which?* magazine in the UK, followed by a spell in the 1980s as a communications specialist with McKinsey & Company in London. She has first degrees in economics (University of Bath) and sociology (Free University Berlin), and in 2003 she completed a doctorate in organisational change at the Business School, University of Hertfordshire. She divides her time between London and rural France, and can be contacted at alidonaldson@gmail.com.

**Elizabeth Lank** is an independent expert in collaborative working. She believes that unconnected organisational silos and poor working relationships account for some of the greatest hidden costs in organisational life – whether in terms of tangible cost and duplication of effort or the wasteful inability to make full use of available human talent. She works with organisations as a coach and advisor to address collaborative working issues and frequently contributes to leadership development programmes on the topic. A graduate of Mount Holyoke College and INSEAD business school, she has published two other books on collaboration and organisational learning. She is based in the UK and can be contacted at elizabeth.lank@think.plus.com.

**Jane Maher** has been a consultant oncologist in the UK's National Health Service (NHS) for nearly 25 years, after training at London and Harvard Universities. She is the Medical Director of an award-winning cancer support and information service (the Lynda Jackson Macmillan Centre in Hertfordshire, England), holds honorary academic appointments at University College London and the Business School, University of Hertfordshire and has published over 100 peer-reviewed publications. For the last 10 years, she has also worked as Chief Medical Officer with the UK charity Macmillan Cancer Support (which celebrates its centenary in 2011) and as a National Clinical Lead with NHS Improvement. She has a longstanding interest in exploring ways to harness the energy of both professionals and lay people to support the improvement of services for people with cancer. She can be contacted at jmaher@macmillan.org.uk.

# Acknowledgements

A big thank you first of all to all the members of the communities of influence described in this book – including dozens of health professionals, researchers, patients and carers. We are particularly grateful to those who gave extra time to helping us write their personal portraits, including Stephen Barclay, Dermott Davison, Bob Grant, Rosie Loftus, Roberta Lovick and Margaret White. Sadly, one of the patient advocates we worked with (Carol Fahey) passed away while we were finishing this book, and we would particularly like to acknowledge the energy she gave to helping others despite living with multiple cancer herself.

Without Macmillan Cancer Support, none of this work would have happened. It was particularly enjoyable to work closely over a prolonged period with Macmillan staff, especially Jim Elliott, Glyn Purland and Lorraine Sloan (who carries on good work with the GP community to this day).

Many others were involved in the work at various stages and helped us piece together a story spanning nearly two decades: special thanks to Jane Bradburn, Judy Young, Cherry Mackie, Beverley Roberts, Lisa Godfrey, Liz Rowett, Melanie Ripley and Heather Monteverde.

A few close colleagues, especially Patricia Shaw, Theodore Taptiklis and Richard Wetenhall, were generous enough to plough through drafts, and the book is almost certainly more readable as a result of their frank and thoughtful suggestions.

Thanks also to Gillian Nineham at Radcliffe Publishing for her incisive comments in the earlier stages of writing, which helped us to shape the book for a broader audience.

Going back even further, other friends and colleagues played their own parts in the making of this book. John Shotter, a prolific author himself, looked at the two green loose-leaf folders containing some 30 narrative accounts accumulated over three years and said 'surely something could be done with all this material'.

Finally we would like to thank each other. We have now been enjoying a productive collaboration for seven years and continue to find new and exciting projects to tackle together. By all accounts, few people are as lucky as we have been in co-authoring a book without falling out even once.

# List of abbreviations

| | |
|---|---|
| GP | General Practitioner |
| GPA | Macmillan GP Advisor |
| MSP | The Macmillan Support Programme for PCCLs in the NHS |
| NHS | National Health Service |
| NURG | National User Reference Group sponsored by Macmillan Cancer Support as part of the National Cancer Genetics Pilots Programme |
| PCT | primary care trust |
| PCCL | Primary Care Cancer Lead |
| RCGP | Royal College of General Practitioners |
| SIL | Service Improvement Lead |
| SDM | Macmillan Service Development Manager |

# Introduction: A fresh approach to improving services

## Encouraging change from the ground up

### OVERVIEW

*For many years, there has been a groundswell of frustration in the UK and elsewhere with top-down, bureaucratic control, especially in the public sector. While we aren't suggesting that management or measurement should stop, the experiences described in this book have convinced us that 'communities of influence' offer a fresh way of thinking about change and service improvement, and that they can contribute to sustainable large-scale change in healthcare and beyond.*

This book is essentially about the value of working relationships that do not appear on organisation charts – but often outlast formal structures. With *Communities of Influence*, we are attempting to show what is possible when groups of people, whether in their capacity as professional practitioners or as members of the public, meet regularly to exchange experiences and have an influence in a particular field.

A number of developments make this subject topical today. In recent times there has been considerable interest in 'communities of practice' but relatively little empirical, longitudinal evidence about them. For a number of years, we (the authors) have been tracking the evolution of a number of communities and groups in the UK health sector, mainly made up of doctors or patients, who want to make a difference to cancer care. *Communities of Influence* takes the communities-of-practice discussion in a new direction: what if you want to create a particular group (professional or lay) not just to share knowledge (as a community of practice does) but also to *influence practice and policy*? How are communities of influence best created and sustained? And is it possible to trace their influence over time?

## FRUSTRATIONS WITH MANAGERIALISM

The way of working described here contrasts with (but can complement) the managerial and bureaucratic approaches prevalent today, such as performance management, centrally-defined targets and evidence-based guidelines. Rather than relying solely on these methods, working through people in groups means taking conversations and relationships seriously. One of our premises is that health professionals, by and large, want to provide good care to patients, like to share knowledge and experience with their peers and want to be able to influence and improve the complex healthcare system around them.

We are not the only authors inquiring into how to influence in a complex world. Others have argued that, in today's environment, leaders and managers should pay more attention to the informal, conversational or 'organic' aspects of organisational life. Like us, they draw inspiration from complexity thinking, arguing that organisational change emerges from countless informal conversations and everyday interactions. For example, in *Informal Coalitions*, Chris Rodgers emphasises the 'messy, informal and a-rational dynamics of organizational change', and goes on to explain how managers can 'act politically, with integrity', by building informal coalitions of support for new ideas.[1] Similarly, in *Unmanaging*, Theodore Taptiklis describes an initiative that began around 2002, engaging groups of professionals in capturing and sharing their daily working experience. This work led him to emphasise the importance of storytelling and to urge us all to recognise ourselves as social beings.[2]

*Communities of Influence* is not an anti-management book. We accept that structures, strategies and procedures are necessary in modern organisations. But there is immense potential for people to become more skilled at working through networks, relationships and conversations to achieve their objectives. In the first place, managers are increasingly recognising the importance of *getting better at engaging people* rather than attempting to control them – to work in partnership with them rather than just giving directions. This is vital because, if professionals find they are being over-managed or not getting what they want from their work, they are likely to vote with their feet. This is as true of line management structures – where jobs are no longer for life – as it is of working in communities.

By learning how to work with communities of influence, managers and other practitioners can also *develop a better understanding of the nature of learning, change and influence*. In a world that seems increasingly complex, unpredictable and uncontrollable, many people feel uncertain about how they can make a difference. They know that learning does not come solely through manuals, guidelines or databases, and they see that written plans, strategies and programmes are insufficient and seldom bring about the change promised. Often what looked good on paper fails to be implemented on the ground.

Encouragingly, we do have evidence that members of the communities of influence described in the next few chapters have made a difference – by sharing their experiences, making useful connections, developing a collective voice and influencing policymakers.

#### Potential contribution of voluntary organisations

The book also provides a case study of how a voluntary organisation has influenced and improved public services, by reaching beyond its own boundaries and engaging with both professionals and lay people. The main sponsor and funder of the work described is the UK charity Macmillan Cancer Support (we say more about Macmillan in Chapter 1). Voluntary organisations have long been in a strong position, given their enthusiasm and autonomy, to act as a force for change. They are central to the notion of the 'Big Society' championed by the UK government in 2010, and even if that phrase becomes 'old hat' with the eventual passing of that government, the aims are likely to remain relevant, namely 'to create a climate that empowers local people and communities, building a big society that will take power away from politicians and give it to people'.[3] The idea is certainly worth exploring further, as one respected UK think tank has said:

> *For some, the coalition government's central idea – the Big Society – is a polite way of saying the 'small state', or simply a way of trying to distract the public from dramatic spending cuts. For others – including the RSA – it is as yet an unformed but nonetheless potentially interesting idea that could place civic action and citizen empowerment centre stage in British politics. (Royal Society for the encouragement of Arts, Manufactures and Commerce)*[4]

The problem with phrases like 'citizen empowerment' or a 'new kind of conversation between government, public services and members of the public' is that they are rather global and relatively meaningless until people work out together what they mean in practice and in detail. *Communities of Influence* provides some concrete examples of how this might look in the real world – health professionals sharing knowledge and ideas, doctors engaging with policymakers, and service developers collaborating with academics (or even being academics themselves).

## CONTRIBUTING TO LARGE-SCALE CHANGE

In this book we give many examples of how communities of influence have contributed to change in a more 'bottom-up' way than is usual in either public services or business. But can this way of working contribute to large-scale change, and how does this compare to what others have written about this topic? Below we look briefly at two bodies of knowledge that have influenced public services: social movement theory and service improvement methodologies.

### Social movements

About five years ago, the UK's National Health Service funded a review of the 'social movements literature' and its implications for large-scale change in the NHS.[5] In *Towards a Million Change Agents*, Bate *et al.* noted that social movements tend to mobilise around a shared grievance – well-known examples include: peace movements, religious movements, civil rights and pro-democracy movements, the labour movement, women's movements, gay and lesbian rights movements, environmental movements and fascist movements.

People working on Barack Obama's successful 2008 presidential election campaign employed many of the principles of social movement theory and this may have helped win over local communities. However, as Bate, *et al.* noted, no one can predict the emergence of movements, make them happen or consciously construct them. And certainly no one can fully control their direction and impact.[6] Indeed, we think there are major risks in adopting this approach to change. One of these is that the high expectations generated among people will almost inevitably be disappointed over time as politicians fail to deliver on many if not most of their promises. While it makes sense to appeal to people's hearts as well as their minds, and tap into their hopes about the future, a backlash seems almost unavoidable at some stage.

The context for the social movement review mentioned above was that, in 2000, the NHS had published ambitious plans for improvement in healthcare.[7] So, at that time there was pressure to understand how large-scale change happened and what, if anything, the UK government and NHS leaders could do to generate it. The 'NHS improvement revolution' was to be delivered by means of dozens of national programmes, coordinated by the then NHS Modernisation Agency. The programmes were to tackle priority areas such as cancer, heart disease and mental health services. Some success, particularly in reducing waiting times for patients, was achieved. However, Bate *et al.* found that there was widespread agreement among experts that most organisations attempting such large-scale change efforts were left with disappointing results. Surveys suggested that most people at the front line of patient care thought that the NHS's programmatic approach to change would not be sufficient to 'achieve our vision of organisation-wide modernisation within the timescales set'.[8]

Most pertinent to our topic is Bate, *et al.*'s conclusion that large-scale change in organisations depends on the 'ability to connect with and mobilise people's own internal energies and drivers for change, in so doing, creating a bottom-up, locally led, grass-roots movement for improvement and change'.[9] Interestingly for this book Bate *et al.* refer to *communities of practice* as 'near movements', explaining that they 'just fall short of that elusive phenomenon of a movement, where people are fired into taking action collectively and the process acquires its own energy and momentum'.[10]

Social movements have a lot in common with communities of influence – for example, the emphasis on relationships over time. A key difference, however, is that those who set up the communities of influence described in this book were not trying to win a short-term campaign or creating unrealistic expectations.

### Service improvement methodologies

Many people have developed models specifically to help organisations tackle the complex challenges of improving services in healthcare. For example, according to the Institute for Healthcare Improvement (IHI) in the USA, the best way to improve care is to conduct small, local tests, using Plan-Do-Study-Act (PDSA) cycles, in which people learn from taking action.[11] With respect to large-scale change, IHI has developed a model called 'Framework for Spread', which suggests some general areas to consider as a large-spread project is undertaken (including leadership, identification of ideas, communication, strengthening of the social system, measurement and feedback).[12] None of these models conflict with the notion of working with communities of influence. However, like all models, they are simplifications of lived experience. In our work, rather than developing such models, we have chosen to focus on what it takes to work through people and long-term relationships.

Another US author, Paul Plsek, looking at how innovation works in healthcare, has distinguished three interrelated processes: generation, implementation, and widespread adoption of ideas.[13] Significantly, he goes on to say that spread is 'primarily an issue of knowledge sharing through social networks', which very much accords with the subject of this book. What his conceptual distinctions do remind us of is that there is often no shortage of ideas for improvement – the hardest part is implementing them. And implementation often fails on account of contextual factors such as inadequate systems and processes or power issues. Another common mistake is trying to spread new ideas before they have been tested locally.

### Communities are not change programmes

Finally, it is worth stressing that the communities we are describing should not be thought of as 'change programmes'. It does not work to apply traditional project management to them, with milestones and deliverables (although communities do often spawn specific projects that can be managed in this way). People get involved because they want to, and may withdraw if they stop seeing any value for themselves in continuing.

The communities-of-influence work described here emerged 'from the ground up', with quite a bit of help from the sponsoring organisation and a number of committed individuals. In the next chapter, we trace back to some of the early seeds of this work, and this takes us on two parallel journeys: the growth of the patient voice in the UK during the 1990s, and the emergence over the same period of a community of GPs dedicated to improving care for people living with cancer.

We do not want this book to create the impression that we are offering an off-the-shelf approach to public service improvement that can be applied anywhere. The danger of presenting the story from a retrospective point of view is that readers may be tempted to throw together their own communities of influence without fully appreciating the importance of history and context. We hope that we have made clear the skill and patience that it takes to develop lively and influential communities.

## MAKING EPHEMERAL ACTIVITIES MORE VISIBLE

One of the challenges in working with communities of influence is that so much of the work consists of conversations and stories, and these can seem ephemeral and intangible to anybody not participating in them directly. *Communities of Influence* therefore takes up the important question of how complex human endeavours are best evaluated. As well as providing evidence for future practice, evaluation plays a vital part in satisfying managers and funders that money has been well spent and is benefiting the people it was intended to help. The writing methods we developed can be described as a form of narrative-based evaluation, and the examples in this book nearly all derive from what we refer to as our 'narrative tracking' work.

### Complexity-informed narrative evaluation

In Chapter 2 we describe our tracking methods in more detail, and compare them with other, similar approaches. They were underpinned by recent thinking on organisational change, particularly complexity thinking.[14,15] In summary, complexity theory helps to explain how change emerges from human interaction, which by its very nature involves power and politics with a small 'p'. For us, it provided discipline to a way of working that may, at first sight, appear unusually informal and unstructured. It included the following:

- Engaging with people to produce an emerging story – as narrative writers we took part in community conversations, listened to people's experiences, produced drafts, discussed these with members, and revised them repeatedly to incorporate new information and stories that emerged. In this way, the accounts had a strong authorial hand yet they were, to a significant extent, the product of many people and many conversations.

- Always seeking to stimulate further reflection and sensemaking,[16] not to produce documentation for its own sake.
- Reflecting complex causality in the narrative accounts, which included avoiding oversimplified 'a led to b' claims, being mindful of the non-linearity of change and paying attention to experience.

## FINDING YOUR WAY AROUND *COMMUNITIES OF INFLUENCE*

Chapter 1, 'The power of the collective voice', introduces Macmillan Cancer Support and explains how a charity best known for its nurses also came to work with doctors in order to improve care for people living with cancer. We also show how this work was informed and inspired by early experiences with patient self-help groups.

Chapter 2, 'Making the invisible visible', takes up the crucial question of how to evaluate this kind of complex endeavour. It lays out the narrative writing methods we developed to enable those not directly involved in community conversations to see more clearly what difference they made. This 'narrative tracking' is the source of many of the later case-study chapters in this book (Chapters 3, 5 and 7), which provide rare long-term empirical evidence of healthcare improvements coming about through collective effort.

Chapter 3, 'Working with and through doctors', is the first of the case-study chapters, telling the story of a community of influence made up of professionals from one discipline – in this case GPs – and what it accomplished over time.

Chapter 4, 'The social life of documents', takes up a particular aspect of community impact: how to increase the chances that the written products often created by groups, such as guidelines for good practice, succeed in influencing behaviour, rather than merely gathering dust.

Chapter 5, 'Hybrid creatures', is the second case-study chapter and tells the story of a group of professionals of combined identities – mainly university researchers with clinical backgrounds – who developed the knowledge and evidence needed to improve services. Their multiple identities put them in a strong position to influence research, education and services on the ground.

Next, for those keen to know what kind of resources and skills are involved in sustaining communities of influence, Chapter 6, 'Cultivating a lively community', describes the vital role of the 'supporting team'. With each Macmillan-sponsored community, this team included different combinations of the following: community sponsor, community facilitator, skilled administrator and clinical lead.

Chapter 7, 'Involving lay people as partners', takes a closer look at the role of patients and carers in communities of influence. Macmillan invited patients and carers into its GP community, but it also worked with dedicated groups of people living with cancer to help improve services.

Finally, in Chapter 8, 'Playing a long game', we flag further insights and questions that have arisen for us as we have worked on this book. It is our hope that by sharing our experience, we will enable others to understand how communities of influence emerge and what kind of support they need to make a difference in a chosen sphere.

## NOTES


1 Rodgers C. *Informal Coalitions: mastering the hidden dynamics of organizational change.* Basingstoke: Palgrave Macmillan; 2006.
2 Taptiklis T. *Unmanaging: opening up the organization to its own unspoken knowledge.* Basingstoke: Palgrave Macmillan; 2008.
3 www.number10.gov.uk/news/latest-news/2010/05/big-society-50248 (accessed 23 December 2010).
4 www.thersa.org (accessed 23 December 2010).
5 Bate P, Bevan H, Robert G. *Towards a Million Change Agents: a review of the social movements literature – implications for large-scale change in the NHS.* London: NHS Modernisation Agency; 2005. Available at: www.library.nhs.uk/Improvement/ViewResource.aspx?resID=325326 (accessed 23 February 2011).
6 Ibid. p. 44.
7 Department of Health. *The NHS Plan: a plan for investment, a plan for reform.* London: Department of Health – Crown Copyright; 2000.
8 Bate, *et al.* op. cit. p. 7.
9 Ibid.
10 Ibid. p. 4.
11 Berwick D. Developing and testing changes in delivery of care. *Annals of Internal Medicine.* 1998; **128**(8): 651–6. See also www.ihi.org (accessed 23 February 2011).
12 Ibid.
13 Plsek P. Complexity and the adoption of innovation in health care. *Conference paper: Accelerating quality improvement in health care – strategies to speed the diffusion of evidence-based innovations;* 2003 January 27–28; Washington, DC. Available at: http://74.125.155.132/scholar?q=cache:MS45tOwCYzMJ:scholar.google.com/+Plsek+Complexity+and+the+adoption+of+innovation+in+health+care&hl=en&as_sdt=2000&as_vis=1 (accessed 23 February 2011).
14 Shaw P. *Changing Conversations in Organizations: a complexity approach to change.* London: Routledge; 2002.

15 Stacey R. *Experiencing Emergence in Organizations: local interaction and the emergence of global pattern.* London: Routledge; 2005.

16 The term 'sensemaking' is widespread in writings on organisational change and communication – see for example: Weick K. *Sensemaking in Organizations.* London: SAGE Publications; 1995; and Dervin B, Foreman-Wernet L, with Lauterbach E. *Sense-Making Methodology Reader.* New Jersey: Hampton Press; 2003. It refers to the way in which we explain or 'make sense of' what happens and what people tell us. It is dialogical (conversational) and can therefore be contrasted with the 'transmission model of communication', which refers to 'the traditional way of talking and thinking about communication whereby the sender sends a message through a communication channel to a receiver' (Dervin *et al.*, op.cit. p. 5).

CHAPTER 1

# The power of the collective voice

## How a charity known for its nurses came to work with general practitioners

### OVERVIEW

*To understand how the idea of communities of influence came about, we need to trace back to what was happening in the 1990s in the UK. Our story follows two parallel developments: in one, a charity best known for its nurses started working with doctors and managed to develop a nationwide 'GP community' dedicated to improving cancer care; meanwhile, the UK was experiencing a surge in patient involvement, and the insights from some research into self-help groups created by cancer patients provided some of the inspiration for working with groups of doctors.*

*It was only much later, in 2008, that we found ourselves coining the phrase 'communities of influence'. What has become apparent is that this way of working through people in groups offers an important opportunity to anybody seeking to improve services in the health sector and beyond.*

The main sponsor and funder of the work described in this book is a charitable organisation that is a household name in the UK – Macmillan Cancer Support (referred to throughout this book as 'the sponsoring organisation' or 'the funding organisation'). Founded back in 1911 as a 'society for prevention and relief of cancer', Macmillan subsequently came to be associated particularly with its 'Macmillan nurses', the first of whom were appointed in 1975 to help patients cope with the symptoms associated with cancer and its treatment. At the time of writing there were more than 3000 Macmillan nurses across the UK. These nursing posts are funded for three years by Macmillan, after which the NHS typically takes on their funding. For patients, Macmillan nurses are free of charge and are 'a valued and trusted source of expert information, advice and support'.[1]

## WHY A VOLUNTARY ORGANISATION CHOSE TO WORK WITH DOCTORS

The roots of the Macmillan GP story go back to the 1970s and 1980s, when the hospice movement was growing in the UK. Around this time, it became clear that GPs (family doctors) were struggling to provide cancer patients with the care they needed outside hospital. It was hard for them to develop and maintain the necessary skills, given that they had many other competing work commitments. Cancer had come to be seen as a specialist area involving chemotherapy, radiotherapy and surgery, and even palliative care itself seemed to be turning into another medical specialty. Often GPs felt excluded from the care of dying patients. As one GP who played a key part in this story told us: 'It was almost taken out of your hands'.

In 1989, Macmillan therefore approached the body responsible for training GPs, the Royal College of General Practitioners (RCGP), to see what could be done to engage GPs in improving the experience of people affected by cancer. The individual who fielded Macmillan's enquiry was himself a GP whose personal experience had given him a keen sense of what was needed:

> *My father's mother had died of stomach cancer when he was 17 and the story he told me of how she died wasn't pleasant. So whenever I managed a dying patient, I did my very best. And there were several occasions when I couldn't do my very best because I didn't know how to; I didn't have enough knowledge or experience. . . . So I said to myself, 'I've got to do something about learning for myself and changing things'. (Ivan Cox)*

He explained how a new approach to educating GPs emerged:

> *Jennifer Raiman (Macmillan's Medical Services Director) had done some research on GPs, which found that they were pretty awful at palliative care. She came and challenged the RCGP, and the chairman passed her letter on to me. So in late 1989 we all sat down together and asked 'What are we going to do about this?', and there were subsequent meetings through January–February 1990 (as with all these things, nothing ever comes of one meeting). (Ivan Cox)*

This description of change emerging through a series of specific conversations is very pertinent to our story, because it reflects one of our fundamental premises

– namely that change emerges from people talking to each other (conversation or dialogue), not just from plans and programmes. It took another two years of meetings and written proposals before all the parties concerned were ready to act. But finally, in 1992, the RCGP General Practice Palliative Care Facilitator Project was launched. In essence, this offered 'protected time' (funded by Macmillan) to six GPs with experience of or an interest in palliative care, releasing them from their clinical responsibilities typically for one day a week. These individuals were based in different parts of the UK and remained practising GPs employed by the NHS, but they could use their protected time to develop their own skills, raise awareness about cancer and palliative care, and provide education, advice and support for other GPs. In addition, they could take steps to improve collaboration with hospitals and specialist palliative care providers (e.g. local hospices). The GPs chosen were known as Macmillan GP Facilitators, but throughout this book we refer to them simply as 'Macmillan GPs'.

It was during these early years that the 'practice visit' became established, whereby Macmillan GPs travelled around discussing palliative and supportive care with primary care teams in their area. They also developed educational material on controlling symptoms and communicating with patients, and they helped compile cancer and palliative care registers and directories of local services.[2] Following the pilot phase, in 1994 Macmillan and the Department of Health agreed to 'roll out' the programme by establishing GP Facilitators across the UK.

As the community began to grow, Jennifer Raiman argued that Macmillan should also appoint 'GP Advisors' (GPAs), who would work closely with the funding organisation and keep in touch with the growing number of GP Facilitators on the ground. The idea was that this would increase Macmillan's ability to influence the national debate on cancer care. In 1994, following further discussions with the RCGP, two Macmillan GP Advisors were appointed (David Millar and Ivan Cox). Their funding covered two days a week each plus administrative support. For the next five years, they travelled the UK recruiting and educating Macmillan GPs.

The GPs were 'Macmillan-badged'. After their Macmillan-funded protected time came to an end (typically it lasted three years), many found local funding to continue the work, but they continued to refer to themselves as 'Macmillan GPs' and remained connected with the charity and its GP community.

### Early evaluations of the Macmillan GP community

Early evaluations gave a sense of the wide-ranging activities pursued by Macmillan GPs in the first decade. One study showed that activity reflected different local contexts and preferences. Much was educational, including courses on topics like 'basics of palliative care' and multidisciplinary meetings on 'breaking bad news'. A key element was visits to other practices, enabling Macmillan GPs to hear about problems faced by their peers and to help them find solutions. Networking with fellow professionals and working on guidelines were also common.[3]

Moreover, relationships between the GPs and their specialist palliative care colleagues had improved, making it easier for GPs to access specialist knowledge. This 'bridge-building' was seen as crucial, because one of the main barriers to continuity and quality of care had been poor relationships between GPs and their colleagues in hospitals.[4]

Another evaluation, undertaken in Wales between 1999 and 2002, found that each of the 17 Macmillan GPs interviewed 'had added substantially to their knowledge and experience of palliative care and palliative care education, the majority to the extent of successfully completing a university diploma in palliative medicine'.[5] Moreover, the very existence of Macmillan palliative care GPs in Wales 'had brought the issue of palliative care into the spotlight'.[6]

An article published by two Macmillan GPs in the journal *Palliative Care Today* in 2001 gave tangible examples of the ripple effects of the community, e.g. a debriefing for a troubled district nurse following the care of a dying child; round-table discussions with two neighbouring hospices who had not talked for 10 years; an increase in appropriate referrals from practices; and gentle support given to a burnt-out GP encountered on a routine visit.[7]

Macmillan's sponsorship enabled the Macmillan GPs to meet one another not just through practice visits but also at community meetings (they gathered regularly as a group from the beginning), where they could share stories, problems and solutions with one other, develop collaborative projects and work out how to influence healthcare policy. These ways of working were in a sense natural to doctors – it was they themselves who pointed out that 'GPs only listen to other GPs'.

## HOW PATIENT GROUPS INSPIRED THE IDEA OF THE 'COLLECTIVE VOICE'

Meanwhile, the early 1990s was also an exciting time for self-help groups and patient involvement.[8] One particular hive of activity emerged at a cancer centre in a hospital in southeast England, and as we shall see, the insights that emerged about developing a 'collective voice' provided important inspiration for Macmillan's continuing work with doctors.

### 'It all began with a row'

One day in the early 1990s, two women met at an event at the Royal Society of Medicine in London, where they were both speakers. One was Jane Maher (a consultant oncologist and co-author of this book), the other was Jane Bradburn, an expert on self-help groups. (For sake of brevity, we will refer to them in this chapter as Jane M and Jane B.) This is how Jane B recalled the encounter with Jane M:

> *I remember quite clearly a person came up to me, and I hadn't experienced her before; she came full-on and said 'It's all very well, these self-help groups, but you don't know what they might be doing. You need somebody to check them out'. (Jane Bradburn)*

'It's not like that,' Jane B retorted, 'the groups set themselves up to meet their own needs'. A lively discussion followed and eventually, Jane M was convinced enough to say 'I think I need to employ you as a patient advocate – come and show me that self-help groups are not full of middle-class women with too much time on their hands'. She wanted to find out why some of her patients were telling her they found self-help groups helpful.

Following this encounter, Jane B embarked on a three-month review of all the self-help groups in the catchment area of the cancer centre at the Mount Vernon Hospital in Hertfordshire, England – 18 groups in total.[9] As well as establishing what it was about these groups that patients found helpful, the aim was to find out *why professionals were not engaging with them*. The first product of this research was a directory of self-help groups in the area. The various self-help groups wrote their own entries, so it was very much their creation. Furthermore, all who wanted to be included in the directory were included, without any vetting, an unusual move at the time.

Next, the two Janes published their findings in an article called 'Community-based self-help groups: an undervalued resource', consciously choosing a peer-reviewed journal (*Clinical Oncology*) so that health professionals would be more likely to take it seriously.[10] This proved reasonably straightforward because, apart from the fact that Jane M was herself an oncologist, the research addressed the sort of questions that other oncologists were asking about patient groups.

### Early forays into partnership working

It was not long before the two Janes began to engage directly with people from the self-help groups. One of the first was a former cancer patient who started working with Jane B as a volunteer (Cherry Mackie).

Another protagonist in this story was Judy Young. As a former radiographer who had worked her way up to become a manager of an NHS cancer centre, she had then trained as a counsellor and set up the counselling service at the Mount Vernon Cancer Centre. So she was what we think of as a 'hybrid creature', which gave her considerable credibility with the medical community. She recalled how challenging she found the early attempts at partnership working:

*I clearly remember the first meeting we had at Mount Vernon with the professionals and the patients. We had invited a particular consultant oncologist onto the organising committee as she was quite anti patient involvement and failed to see the need for any of the psychosocial stuff that we were undertaking. The first meeting was quite difficult. There were about 10 people and the professionals sat on one side of the room while the patients were on the other. I do remember feeling fairly defensive at first, but the more meetings we had the easier it became. (Judy Young)*

Another event followed at Mount Vernon, but this time all the self-help groups set up stalls in a hall and the health professionals came along to find out what they did. Then, over a two-year period, Jane B and Judy co-led a patient and professional working group, meeting self-help groups and listening to their views about what new services could be set up to meet their needs.

### The 'patient voice' helps to shape a brand new service

A key outcome of all their work was a proposal for a new form of support service, designed according to priorities articulated by patients themselves. First, the patients wanted a building where they would be greeted by non-professionals with time to listen to their concerns. Second, they wanted better information. And third, they wanted access to counselling and complementary therapy (oncologists felt particularly challenged by the latter). All these requests were taken into account, and a set of guidelines was drawn up for identification, training and practice of therapists, with a programme of research to demonstrate value. A proposal was duly presented to the executive of the hospital and Macmillan Cancer Support, and the centre was opened at Mount Vernon Hospital in 1993. Judy became the manager of the centre and Cherry Mackie also took on a paid role. (Seventeen years later, Judy had retired but Cherry was still working at the centre in the position of Complementary Therapy and Support Groups Coordinator.)

Crucial support for the new centre came not only from Macmillan but also from the Lynda Jackson family and from Mount Vernon's visionary Chief Executive, Stephen Ramsden, who had always wanted to see a complementary therapy centre at the hospital. The Lynda Jackson Macmillan Centre (LJMC), as it later came to be known, was the first support and information unit based in a major cancer centre and designed around priorities expressed by patients. Much of the thinking found its way into the 2000 Cancer Plan for England as an example of good practice. By 2007, no less than 60 similar centres had opened in the UK and Australia.[11] Significantly for our communities of influence story, the LJMC demonstrated the power of the collective voice of cancer patients to make a difference.

### Perspectives combined to create new guidance on communication

Meanwhile, Jane B had set up a patient involvement research unit at Mount Vernon. The first study undertaken was based on a declared patient priority: how health professionals delivered bad news. It involved focus groups with members of support groups and interviews with 27 consultants and culminated in a report (*Breaking Bad News*), published by the Kings Fund in 1996.[12] What was special about this publication was that the issue was looked at from both the clinician's and the patient's point of view, in order to find answers that met the needs of each party to the communication.

Though *Breaking Bad News* turned out to be one of the Kings Fund's bestsellers (and was still in print in 2010), the auditable guidelines contained in it were not fully implemented. This was an early lesson showing that, although it is important to create guidelines, they can only change behaviour if the ground is well prepared, e.g. if people work together to identify what needs to happen to make implementation possible. In other words, it is crucial to give the guidelines a 'social life' in order to test whether they are likely to influence behaviour.

### 'Cancer Voices' emerge

All the work at Mount Vernon described so far contained seeds that later developed into patients having a say in other parts of the NHS. Partnership working received

#### Key lessons about enabling patients to work with professionals

*Lay people benefit from having time together to 'find their voice':* This gave them the confidence needed to mingle with health professionals.

*Experiential knowledge counts:* Effort had to go into persuading health professionals to take 'experiential knowledge' seriously, but ultimately the stories and ideas that came out of *groups* came to be seen as more reliable than those that came from *individuals*.

*Emphasis may shift over time:* Over time, people in self-help groups 'moved from support to influence'; in other words, initially some needed to 'get their needs met', but later many moved on to become patient advocates.

*It can be vital to pay attention to detail:* It was not enough just to say to professionals 'all your work should involve lay people'. For partnership working to be viable, somebody had to pay attention to detail (e.g. make sure people's travel expenses were reimbursed).

*Publishing makes a difference:* In a medical environment, writing up and publishing the findings of the research was vital as a way of demonstrating evidence of the value of working with self-help groups and developing a 'patient voice'.

a boost from publication in 1995 of the Calman Hine report on the future of cancer services, which anticipated patient involvement in the new cancer networks in the UK.[13]

To support and train patients for this work Jane B set up an action research project at Mount Vernon, and in 1999 she went to work with UK charity Cancer Link to develop similar work on a national basis, by setting up the Cancer Voices project. This created a trained and supported network of people working to improve cancer services, and Jane B later published an account of how the early work with self-help groups informed national developments.[14] (Cancer Voices will crop up again in our story – *see* Chapter 7.)

A number of insights emerged from all this pioneering work with patients and carers (*see* box).

## AMPLIFYING THE VOICE OF THE GP COMMUNITY

Resuming the Macmillan GP story started earlier, Jane Maher was seconded by the NHS to take up the role of Chief Medical Officer at Macmillan on a part-time basis in 1999. This made her responsible for engaging doctors as part of the charity's work as a 'force for change' in the field of cancer and supportive care. From the start, Jane was convinced of the power of groups – inspired to some extent by the research into self-help groups in Hertfordshire. She asked herself: 'If we have effective, influential patient groups, why couldn't we do something similar with GPs?' Just as patients needed confidence to work with professionals, GPs needed to be able to engage with specialist doctors and NHS decision-makers with influence and authority.

Though herself a specialist consultant doctor, Jane was particularly keen to strengthen the voice of the GP in cancer care. The GP was, after all, usually the first professional consulted by a person with possible cancer symptoms. Moreover, within the medical profession, family doctors were the ones most able to relate to their patients as whole people – rather than focusing on a specific illness, they could form a picture of how all the illnesses added up together. Indeed, the UK can be seen as fortunate in having GPs and other general practice staff to care for cancer patients in the community. (Family doctors in the USA, for example, have a much less prominent role in healthcare, particularly in the diagnosis of cancer.) Significantly for Macmillan, its own nurses, who were often the ones associated with caring for cancer patients at home, agreed that the GP was a key player in the field of supportive care.

The growing community of Macmillan GPs was also a way for Macmillan as an organisation to engage with and influence GPs. This was seen as hard for it to do. Why? First, there was no 'typical GP' and they were spread across the country in thousands of GP practices. Second, as generalists, on any normal working day they saw myriad symptoms and illnesses that might or might not have anything to do with cancer. Third, with other chronic illnesses such as diabetes and heart disease, some GPs felt they had more control of the treatment than they did with cancer, which was seen as 'an acute sector illness'. On the other hand, GPs were typically self-motivated and, once engaged, willing to do more than was asked of them.

### 'Bottom-up influence'

Ideas and stories shared in GP community meetings were constantly subjected to testing by peers, enabling a 'collective voice' to emerge. This made it easier for the GPs as a group to influence healthcare policies, and many recent improvements in cancer and supportive care in the UK can be traced back to conversations in the Macmillan GP community over the past two decades.

The focus of the first few years was on how best to care for dying patients – an issue that all GPs tend to be confronted with in their practice. One of the earliest specific problems tackled by the GPs was what to do about cancer patients who suddenly need a doctor when their local general practice was closed or unavailable (e.g. during the night, at the weekend or on a public holiday) – the 'out-of-hours' problem.[15] In Chapter 3, 'Working with and through doctors', we give many more examples of advances in care that emerged from the Macmillan GP community.

There was learning in all this for Macmillan as a sponsoring organisation: acting as a force for change was not just about high-level campaigning, but also about 'bottom-up influence'. And despite a perception by some that GPs' time was expensive to buy, the reality was that the charity only had to provide GPs with one day a week of protected time to enable them to pursue their educational and influencing activities.

By the mid 2000s, there were some 100 Macmillan GPs and they were increasingly seen (or rather heard) as a respected collective voice by Macmillan and NHS policymakers. They made up a community that was essentially 'uni-disciplinary', i.e. just included GPs. Experience had shown that any given group (e.g. doctors, nurses, patients) was best able to develop a collective voice when its members had a chance to share experiences and problems among themselves before opening their doors more widely.

### New group spins off existing community

Meanwhile, drawing on some of the lessons learned with the GP community, in 2003 Macmillan set up a small group of clinician researchers ('hybrid creatures' – *see* Chapter 5). Research and evidence were urgently needed to help improve services in end-of-life care and this was a novel way of making sure that academic research influenced services on the ground. Members of this group, some of whom were also members of the GP community, contributed to knowledge and evidence and succeeded in attracting extra funding for studies in this important but under-researched field.

In addition to these professional groups (the GPs and the clinician researchers), Macmillan worked directly with people living with cancer (*see* Chapter 7).

Thus, over time, a whole range of groups and communities of influence emerged, most of which are portrayed in this book. In terms of size, they ranged from networks of 100–250 professionals to much smaller groups of around 15 people living with cancer. Whatever their size, the activities of these communities gave the sponsoring organisation far greater reach and influence than it would otherwise have had as a charity with a few hundred employees.

### Communities of influence: a new concept emerges

It was not until 2008 that we (the three co-authors of this book) found ourselves coining the phrase 'communities of influence'. We were all aware of Wenger's publications on 'communities of practice', a term first developed in the context of learning theory.[16] Wenger argued that learning is a fundamentally social phenomenon and that we all belong to and participate in informal communities of practice, in which we refine our practice, negotiate meaning and develop a sense of identity. The following definition of communities of practice seemed to fit the Macmillan-sponsored groups quite well:

> *[G]roups of people who share a concern, a set of problems, or a passion about a topic, and who deepen their knowledge and expertise in this area by interacting on an ongoing basis . . .*[17]

However, it struck us that the term 'communities of practice' didn't quite capture the essence of the groups we were working with, the main *raison d'être* of which was to *have an influence* on cancer care. In general, people joined them and stuck with them mainly because they wanted to make a difference to people living with cancer.

### Why not 'network'?

People use various words to refer to groups of people with a shared interest or purpose, such as 'community', 'network' or 'collaborative'. For us, the exact term chosen seemed less important than the idea that it is *relationships, connections and conversations* that matter. Relationships are what makes a community, but they also emerge and grow from community conversations. Furthermore, while the nature and membership of a community can change over time, the relationships formed in it can go on for years – and outlive more formal organisational structures.

### Opportunities beyond cancer care

There are many parts of the health sector that might make use of communities of influence as a way of working through people to improve services. The growth of chronic conditions is one obvious starting place. Of around 500 000 deaths in England each year, the majority occur following a period of chronic illness related to conditions such as heart disease, diabetes, cancer, stroke, dementia, liver, renal, neurological and chronic respiratory diseases.[18] Indeed, while we were writing this book, media commentators were saying 'Alzheimer's is the next cancer'. As this and other chronic conditions become more common in an aging population, there will be value in enabling committed professionals and lay people to share experience, develop a collective voice and influence policymakers.

## BEYOND HEALTHCARE

Indeed, many organisations, not just those concerned with healthcare, depend on people from diverse disciplines or cultures and disparate locations working jointly towards a common purpose – whether they are teachers, engineers, social workers, sales people, IT specialists, clerical workers, volunteers or any other group that shares a professional practice. But there are often serious hurdles to overcome: people may be physically dispersed; may not work for the same employer; and may not even know each other. As a former Chief Executive of Macmillan Cancer Support put it:

> *It's fundamentally about getting different professional groups to work collaboratively and to respect each other. For the Maritime and Coastguard Agency for example, the marine surveyors, the coastguards and the civil servants each have their language, culture and ethical code built up over decades or even centuries. But they share the Agency's common goal of protecting the safety of life at sea and they have to work together to achieve it. (Peter Cardy, then CEO of the Maritime and Coastguard Agency, now CEO of Aquaterra)*

Communication technologies such as email, web forums and teleconferencing can help, but they are no substitute for the trust, confidence and motivation that can grow through regular face-to-face contact.

There is, however, evidence that communities of influence can contribute something to improving services in a complex environment, at a local and national level. This book inquires into what that 'something' is.

## NOTES


1 www.macmillan.org.uk/HowWeCanHelp/Nurses/AboutMacmillanNurses.aspx (accessed 23 December 2010).
2 Millar DG, Carroll D, Grimshaw J, *et al.* Palliative Care at Home: an audit of cancer deaths in the Grampian region. *British Journal of General Practice.* 1998; **48**(431): 1299–302.
3 Shipman C, Thompson M, Pearce A, *et al. Building Bridges: the Macmillan GP facilitator programme in palliative care – an evaluation 1998–2000.* London: Department of Palliative Care & Policy, Kings College London; 2001.
4 Ibid.
5 Clark D, Hughes P, Ingleton C, Noble B. *We didn't know what we didn't know: evaluation of Powys Macmillan General Practitioner Clinical Facilitator Project – final report.* Sheffield: Sheffield Palliative Care Studies Group, University of Sheffield; 2002. p. 37.
6 Ibid. p. 38.
7 Thomas K, Millar D. Catalysts for change – Macmillan GP facilitators in cancer and palliative care. *Palliative Care Today.* 2001; **9**: pp. 54–6.
8 For a summary of self-help activities, as things stood in the mid 1990s, see: Wann M. *Building Social Capital: self-help in a twenty-first century welfare state.* London: Institute for Public Policy Research; 1995.
9 Mount Vernon Cancer Centre serves a population of 2 000 000. Annually, 5000 new cancer patients are referred to 25 oncology consultants, with oncologists visiting 12 district general hospitals and liaising with more than 100 surgeons and physicians and with 10 000 primary care physicians and community nurses. See Maher EJ. An integrated support and information centre in a large UK cancer centre established in 1993 and replicated in more than 60 units across the United Kingdom and Australia. *Current Oncology.* 2008; **15**(Suppl. 2).
10 Bradburn J, Maher EJ, Young J, *et al.* Community-based self-help groups: an undervalued resource. *Clinical Oncology.* 1992; **4**: 377–80.
11 Maher, op. cit.
12 Walder G, Bradburn J, Maher J. *Breaking Bad News.* London: Kings Fund; 1996.
13 www.cancer.nhs.uk/ and www.dh.gov.uk/en/Publicationsandstatistics/Publications/PublicationsPolicyAndGuidance/Browsable/DH_4992540 (accessed 23 February 2011). The Calman/Hine Report, published in 1995, recommended cancer networks as the organisational model for cancer services to implement the NHS Cancer Plan. They bring together health service commissioners and providers (primary care and hospitals), the voluntary sector, and local authorities. Each network typically serves a population of around one to two million people.
14 Bradburn J, Mackie T. A foot in the door: a collaborative action research project with cancer service users. In: Munn-Giddings C, Winter R, editors. *A Handbook for Action Research in Health and Social Care.* New York: Routledge; 2001. pp. 187–99.

15 Thomas K. *Out-of-Hours Palliative Care in the Community: continuing care for the dying at home*. London: Macmillan Cancer Relief; 2001.
16 Wenger E. *Communities of Practice: learning, meaning and identity*. Cambridge: Cambridge University Press; 1998.
17 Wenger E, McDermott R, Snyder W. *Cultivating Communities of Practice: a guide to managing knowledge.* Boston, MA: Harvard Business School Press; 2002.
18 Department of Health. *End of Life Care Strategy: promoting high quality care for all adults at the end of life – executive summary.* July 2008. www.endoflifecareforadults.nhs.uk/assets/downloads/pubs_EoLC_Strategy_exec.pdf (accessed 23 February 2011).

## CHAPTER 2

# Making the invisible visible

## The importance of tracking life and achievements of communities over time

### OVERVIEW

*One of the challenges in working with the Macmillan communities of influence was how to make their activities and achievements more visible, especially for those funding the work. By involving a narrative writer over time, it was possible both to track the evolution and influence of the groups and to use the written accounts to stimulate debate and learning.*

*Over time, the writing took many forms, including group narratives, individual portraits, discussion papers on emerging themes and tabular summaries. We particularly emphasise the power of iterative writing, by which we mean producing successive draft accounts in order to develop a story over time and involve others in the process, thus allowing evaluation and learning to go hand in hand. Finally, academic underpinning was important to the sponsors of this work and our writing was particularly informed by thinking on complexity and emergence. This provided discipline to a way of working that may, at first sight, appear unusually informal and unstructured.*

By their nature, community conversations are ephemeral or evanescent, and those not participating directly in them may struggle to understand what they produce. In particular, the senior managers responsible for community budgets may have real difficulty 'seeing' the results. The *cost* of investing in communities of influence is typically more immediate and visible to them than the *benefits*. Whereas the costs usually appear up front, many of the benefits take months or even years to materialise. So, without some form of credible 'evaluation', continued funding will always be at risk, and much of the learning and relationships jeopardised. Narrative-based evaluation enabled us to track some of the conversations and stories and thus make the work of the communities more visible – hence the title of this chapter.[1]

## WHY DO CONVERSATIONS AND STORIES MATTER?

Conversations and stories are the lifeblood of communities and organisations of all kinds. Anyone who thinks about how humans learn, or how they influence one another, knows how important these forms of communication are. The problem is that conversation is such a normal part of everyday life – in turn stimulating, boring, routine, touching and frustrating – that people seldom stop to think about what a complex and creative process it is. Furthermore, in a world preoccupied with targets, performance, outcomes and productivity, it is easy to underestimate the importance of an aspect of organisational life that is under our noses all the time. Most of the time we don't even give it any thought.

There is a wealth of literature demonstrating that 'talk' is a vital part of organisational life and business, and that learning and novelty emerge from conversation. 'When people come together in organisations to get things done, they talk', wrote Deirdre Boden in her book *The Business of Talk*.[2] Yet meetings are seen by many as a waste of time, and few people get opportunities or take the trouble to study conversation or improve their skills in it. Perhaps part of the explanation is that, in working life, *things* tend to be valued more highly than talk:

> *Our habits of thought and speech tend to blind us to the sheer flowing ubiquity of the communicative dance in which we are all engaged. Instead we focus mainly on the tangible products of conversation – the organizational designs, performance profiles, business models, strategic frameworks, action plans, lists and categories with which we seek to grasp the reified complexities of organizational life and render them 'manageable'. (Patricia Shaw)*[3]

Even academics who study organisational life tend to overlook conversation, and Boden provides a clue as to why:

> *Virtually all organisational studies study events and decisions long after they occur. They depend on interview, or questionnaires, or the residual records of the organisations themselves, losing entirely the dynamism that is such a central feature of all social organisation. (Deirdre Boden)*[4]

In our work with communities of influence, we took conversations seriously. Far from being 'just talk', they can be thought of as a form of 'joint action', which can be characterised as follows:

> *Its overall outcome is not up to any of the individuals concerned in it; it is entirely novel; its outcomes are as if they have 'come out of the blue'. (John Shotter)*[5]

A key element of the conversational life of communities is of course storytelling. The role of stories in organisations has been extensively explored in recent years.[6] In communities of influence, stories can help reveal problems, patterns, and solutions observed and experienced by members. Ideas and stories shared in community meetings are constantly subject to testing by peers, enabling a 'collective voice' to emerge.

The value of stories is not limited to the learning that occurs when they are first told. Each community member will be in contact with a whole range of people beyond the group, and after leaving a community meeting they may pass on stories and insights. Often the people who told their stories at a meeting may have no idea how far these will travel or what influence they will have (how far the ripples will spread).

In this chapter we focus particularly on our narrative accounts about the Macmillan GP community. Wherever possible we point to what the writing brought to light that might otherwise have remained obscure. For Macmillan, the primary purpose of working through communities was to drive up standards in primary care by engaging GPs and people living with cancer. Such objectives are notoriously difficult to measure. The narrative writing offered a qualitative method of documenting outcomes associated with the communities, including examples of both national and local influence. We start the story in 2003, when a conversation began about how Macmillan might go about evaluating its relatively unpublicised work with doctors, known internally as the 'medical strategy'. The purpose of this work, as stated in internal documents, was to contribute to bringing people-centred practice to all doctors treating and caring for cancer patients throughout the UK.

## EVALUATION FOR LEARNING

> *evaluate: vb – 1 to ascertain or set the amount of value of. 2 to judge or assess the worth of. (Collins Concise Dictionary, 21st-century edition)*

At the outset, we had no predefined or agreed idea of what 'evaluation' was going to mean to us. Macmillan had commissioned many such studies before, but these had been costly by nature and had not always proved as useful as hoped. Once the reports had been looked at, they became more or less dormant, to the frustration of both the Macmillan sponsor and the authors themselves.

As we set out on this evaluation journey, our early conversations clarified that what the Macmillan team needed was a way of both making its work with doctors more visible and stimulating organisational learning. It was important to avoid the learning getting 'stuck' with those who were doing the writing. Instead the team wanted to develop an evaluation method that was fit for purpose, by building learning in from the start. This is how the term 'evaluation for learning' came up. The whole point of the exercise was to explore whether by developing a collective voice (in communities of GPs or of people living with cancer) it was possible to improve quality of care.

For the purpose of communication within Macmillan, we used a more official-sounding term: the 'learning framework' (or 'medical strategy learning framework' whenever we wanted to make it clear that it was Macmillan's medical community that we were focusing on). The term proved useful, as it gave us a legitimate 'thing' to point to in conversations with managers. For us 'framework' did not mean, however, that we were creating a simple, prescriptive model (which is often what 'framework' means in management consulting circles). Rather, we thought of ourselves as 'developing a common language' over time, so we could articulate how Macmillan was working with communities of influence and what this work was achieving.

### Developing language that reflects complexity and emergence

The problem is that so much of management and everyday thinking is imbued with assumptions about how organisations work and how change and improvement come about. A different kind of common language started to emerge for us from our earliest conversations, as phrases like 'surfacing the invisible', 'ripple effects', 'narrative tracking' and 'social life of documents' gained currency between us. Such ways of speaking felt more in tune with the work of cultivating communities than everyday managerial phrases like 'demonstrating impact' or 'measuring performance'. It was not that we were dismissing the importance of measuring outcomes – to the contrary, we knew that this was essential in order to 'keep the show on the road'. But it was important to us to find fresh language to escape taken-for-granted thinking and to use words that fully reflected our understanding of how learning and improvement emerge from human interactions.

### Drawing on diverse backgrounds in the team

When we embarked on the task of narrative tracking, we did not go for an off-the-shelf methodology. We think therefore that it is worth sketching out the experience and interests of those involved in the 'learning framework' discussions, as these naturally influenced the way we went about things in the particular context we found ourselves in. We will start with the three authors of this book.

- Alison Donaldson's main professional interest lay in the part played by writing in the conversational life of organisations, and particularly the value of narrative writing. She introduced the phrase 'social life of documents', which became central to the work.
- Elizabeth Lank had long experience of facilitating collaborative working in and across organisations, and was particularly interested in organisational learning processes such as setting up and cultivating communities of practice to encourage knowledge sharing.
- Jane Maher, as Macmillan's Chief Medical Officer, was responsible for the charity's work with doctors, and needed to feel confident that the methods were underpinned by a body of credible academic thinking.

There were also two Macmillan staff members closely involved with the work at the beginning.

- Glyn Purland, a senior manager with Macmillan (since retired), had a long NHS career behind him. As well as being the budget holder for the work, and therefore particularly keen to see results, he understood the spirit and philosophy of communities of influence. He knew, for example, that he was not just a remote commissioner or funder but a vital colleague in all aspects of the work, and that informal conversations and relationships were to be taken seriously.
- Lorraine Sloan, community facilitator for the Macmillan GP community, had a keen interest in continued learning from Macmillan's work with doctors. She had extensive experience and skill in connecting people to improve quality of care and had introduced patient and carer involvement into this work.

Lorraine and Glyn respectively represented the crucial roles of 'community facilitator' and 'organisational sponsor' (*see* Chapter 6 for more on these roles). Together the five of us made up the central team supporting the communities of influence described in this book.

## HELPING A GROUP REFLECT ON ITS PAST AND ITS FUTURE

When we first sat down together, we did not have a 'grand plan'. However we felt confident that, as we spoke to people and discovered what the Macmillan-supported groups were doing, we would be able to identify examples and stories that could make their work more visible. The most urgent thing in 2004 was to work out where to start. The Macmillan team wanted the narrative tracking to help it secure continued support for the communities, yet had almost no experience of working with us (Alison and Elizabeth) as external consultants. At the beginning we therefore agreed to start with a relatively limited piece of work – something 'quick and dirty', as somebody put it – to test how we could work together.

The first story (or case study) we embarked on was that of the Macmillan GP Advisor group. The GP Advisor role went back to the early 1990s, so one advantage of starting with it was that it allowed us to explore and demonstrate important developments and achievements over time in Macmillan's work with doctors. As champion of this work, Jane Maher was personally convinced that the Macmillan GPs had been highly influential in the NHS, both locally and nationally. In particular, it was important to investigate what role they had played in the emergence and spread of two major advances in cancer care: the Gold Standards Framework (GSF) for end-of-life care in the community, and the relatively new role of Primary Care Cancer Lead (PCCL) in the NHS. The team wanted us to speak to each GP Advisor to hear their perspective and then construct an impartial history demonstrating the group's influence over time.

From a pragmatic point of view, the GP Advisor group was a good place to start because we could construct a narrative account by talking to a small number of people – there were just five GP Advisors at that time, compared with about 100 Macmillan GPs in total and many more health professionals in the wider Macmillan family. All current and past GP Advisors were willing to talk about their experiences (one former member of the group afterwards described the process as cathartic). All in all, the time seemed ripe to create this account and use it to stimulate reflection and help the group reorientate itself for the next phase of its work.

**Contents page of our first narrative account**

***'Engaging with influential doctors'***

We (Alison and Elizabeth) began by attending one of the regular meetings of the GP Advisors in May 2004 in London, and also separately speaking to every member of the group, past as well as current. After two months we had a draft narrative which we called 'Engaging with influential doctors'. As the boxed table of contents shows, the account looked specifically at the influence of Macmillan GPs on two major 'service improvements' – the Gold Standards Framework for palliative care in the community, and the new NHS role of Primary Care Cancer Lead.

### Using the writing to stimulate reflection and discussion

We circulated our draft to the group itself and joined their next meeting, in September 2004 in London, during which we jointly reviewed the account and some of the lessons learned so far. This was an important step because, as with most groups, this one had had its share of tensions (though these had not negated its influence). This discussion prompted the GP Advisors to reserve time in their future meetings to reflect on the group's way of working, and to address any difficulties before they escalated.

At the next meeting, in February 2005 near Edinburgh, we led a discussion about the group's future. We also suggested that it would be useful to share 'Engaging with influential doctors' with Macmillan senior management, so they might better understand the work of the group and the value of continuing to invest in it. The GP Advisors seemed anxious about this at first and requested another chance to read the draft with this particular readership in mind. This stimulated a further iteration of the written account.

It is worth pausing here for a moment to notice what can happen when a document is shared with a new set of readers. In this case, the community written about suddenly became more concerned about what the narrative account said when it realised that politically significant figures were going to see it. More generally, this provides a clue about what motivates a group to do more than just skim-read its own story.

### Our first multiperspective narrative

It was this first piece of work that prompted us to experiment with interweaving different perspectives. Members of the group who had lived through the history had divergent ways of making sense of it. For one particularly controversial strand of the story, we therefore set out a chronological list of events that could be accepted by everybody, followed by three personal perspectives (including the community sponsor and two clinical leaders). This enabled each person to express the story in their own way yet also to see how others put it. Some negotiation followed, but in the end there was a rich record that included different ways of making sense of what had happened.

One of the advantages of weaving together a narrative account in this way is that there is no need to reach a completely agreed version. There is therefore less risk that the story will get watered down into a compromise version with all the telling details removed.

### What can a historical account make visible?

Before we set out to write 'Engaging with influential doctors', the group's achievements over the first 10 years had been in danger of vanishing in the mists of time and organisational politics. The narrative account clarified and highlighted what they had accomplished and gave credit to those who had played a part. The GP Advisors themselves appeared to find value in having someone shine a spotlight on their story – the conversations healed some old wounds and prompted reflection on the next stage of its work. And for his part, community sponsor Glyn Purland clearly started to appreciate what he called 'the value of the rear view mirror in enabling us to drive forwards'.

The experience of retracing the history of the GP Advisor group also helped to further crystallise our thinking about the work of 'cultivating communities'. In particular, Jane Maher began to refer to the GP Advisors as a 'distilling-and-connecting group' that could distil the learning from the wider GP community and be a living link between community and funding organisation.

More generally, from both a complexity and a narrative perspective, history is always worth exploring. Nothing in organisational life comes from nowhere, even though attempts at strategic planning, culture change and change management often invite us to think that it is possible to start with a clean slate and rational analysis. By exploring together what has happened, a group can collectively make sense of its past, and in our experience this usually points the way towards some next move or moves.

## SO WHAT? WHAT DIFFERENCE DID THE NARRATIVE TRACKING MAKE?

The purpose of the narrative tracking was to make the nature and achievements of the communities of influence more visible, whether these were tangible products and programmes, or what we refer to as ripple effects – conversations and stories that are passed on from person to person, provoking learning and influence along the way. But what difference did the written accounts make to members of the communities or to the sponsoring organisation? What might *not* have happened if we *hadn't* tracked the communities? For each community, there seems to have been a moment when having a written record became vital in securing continued support and funding (*see* box).

### Turning points associated with the narrative writing

***The GP community***

Our first narrative account told the story of the Macmillan GPs from 1992–2004 and helped those who had been involved to reflect on their joint history, make sense of it (including some uncomfortable memories), and compare views about what had been achieved by whom (*see* Chapter 3). This helped the group move on and clarify what it would focus on in the months ahead. When the funding organisation later asked us to draw on the narrative material and create a review of the effectiveness of the GP Advisors, this made its achievements visible to senior managers and helped to secure continued funding.

***The hybrid research group***

Similarly, with the 'hybrid' research community (*see* Chapter 5), there was a moment about three years into the group's existence when ongoing funding was due for review. By then, we had several narrative accounts of the group's evolution, so it was easy to create a 'log of achievements' (a table covering several pages itemising members' publications, funding secured, promotions, etc.). Again, this helped persuade senior managers to continue funding the group.

***The patient group***

With the group of people living with cancer that was set up to advise Macmillan on its work with doctors, we were told by community facilitator Lorraine Sloan that our narrative account (*see* Chapter 4) allowed community members to 'see their own story in black and white and to realise that their achievements had been noticed and appreciated'. It was important for members to see the fruits of their work, she added; 'Much of the work within the medical strategy is complex and focused on producing longer-term influence, rather than immediate "products". Therefore it is very important to capture and disseminate anything that gives visibility and credibility to our work so far'. (Lorraine Sloan, community facilitator)

## FURTHER CLARIFYING OUR NARRATIVE WRITING METHODS

As well as creating a shared history and stimulating thoughts about the group's next phase, 'Engaging with influential doctors' enabled us to test whether narrative writing could capture complex processes and provide 'evaluation for learning'. In effect, this first account was the pilot for what turned into a longer-term process of narrative tracking. All in all, between 2004 and 2007, some 30 pieces of writing emerged, including group stories, individual portraits and thematic papers. These all helped people visualise what communities of influence did in practice, and what they could contribute to the lives of people living with cancer. We describe next some of the ways of working that emerged as critical for this tracking work.

### Regular conversations within the team

The Macmillan team acted as a kind of steering group that provided Alison and Elizabeth as external consultant-writers with crucial organisational and political context. The team also continuously reviewed the focus of the work and test-read drafts. From 2004 till 2007 the five of us continued to meet for half a day about once a month to discuss what was happening in the communities, the emerging portfolio of narratives, publication plans, ways of sharing the learning, as well as opportunities to create new communities of influence. Between our meetings we stayed in touch via email, telephone and teleconference, or met informally according to need.

The writers were not the only ones keeping an ear open for stories of influence – all members of the team picked up useful information and examples in their everyday conversations at work. By meeting regularly we were able to share what we had heard, feed it into the narrative accounts and agree what actions were emerging as important or necessary.

### Direct participation in community

In order to track the activities of the communities, Alison and Elizabeth took an active part in community meetings, often facilitated the conversations, listened to and recorded people's experiences, produced narrative drafts, discussed these with the relevant group, and revised the accounts to incorporate new stories that emerged.

The direct involvement of writers in community conversations is worth drawing attention to, as it is not necessarily common practice in research, where often the researchers either interview intentionally or observe quietly. Recent thinking on emergence and organisational change had persuaded us that 'not participating' was impossible – one can never 'stand outside' a group and observe it without influencing it. Even if this were possible, it was never our purpose just to observe – we were there to help the communities develop, to stimulate learning and to assist the team in securing ongoing funding for the community work.

### Iterative writing

One of the most crucial phrases to emerge as we worked together was 'iterative writing'. What this meant to us was that we actively sought opportunities to take our drafts back into each community being tracked, to stimulate renewed sharing of experience and further sensemaking. Additional stories and new thinking could then be woven into the evolving narrative account. The discussions also often led to useful next steps for the communities themselves and for the Macmillan team.

It is worth saying a bit more about the practice of iterative writing. Everyone who writes knows that a piece of writing can improve as successive drafts are worked over and comments incorporated. However, in organisational life, the sender–receiver metaphor retains a subtle but firm hold. This taken-for-granted way of thinking means that people frequently overlook the potential of writing to stimulate reflection and learning in both writer and reader. If one stops to think about it for a moment, it becomes apparent that authors do not just write down what they already know. They learn by writing – it forces them to articulate thoughts and stories in a sequential fashion with sufficient precision for the reader to follow the account. Readers may also learn, provided they engage with the written account.

In other words, inviting members of communities of influence to read and reflect on the draft narrative accounts was not just a formality but a way of encouraging collaborative learning and avoiding a situation where the only person to learn from the process of writing was the author.

### The value of using words exactly as spoken

In developing our second narrative account, which was about a group of people living with cancer, we used a small digital recording device for the first time to capture people's exact words. Over the next three years, we were to record several conversations and meetings, and the material captured enabled us to enrich many of the narrative accounts by including people's words as spoken.

Over time, we experimented with how best to use the recordings. Mostly we transcribed only parts (just enough to enable us to weave striking stories or utterances into our account). On one occasion we experimented with transcribing a whole conversation (with a group of carers) and subsequently circulated it among those who had been present. The limited response to this transcription suggested to us that: (i) we would have a better chance of provoking some responses if we requested a 'slot' at one of their later meetings to discuss the text, and (ii) that it might also be better in future to weave spoken words into more-reader-friendly narrative accounts. This is what we did in much of our subsequent writing, always giving community members a chance to see their words in the drafts, and the option of changing, removing or expanding them.

### Building informal alliances

We also thought continuously about how we could spread the word about what the communities were doing and encourage others to try this way of working through people. After the first few months, we therefore convened an informal workshop to share our thinking with a select group of Macmillan managers representing areas like strategy, human resources, knowledge management and user involvement.

It is a curious fact that people often take external publications about their own organisation more seriously than internal reports. Leif Edvinsson, an early champion for organisational learning in the business world, introduced us to the rather apt phrase 'boomerang marketing' to characterise this phenomenon.[7] This notion encouraged us to seek opportunities for publication in peer-reviewed management and medical journals. Our first external publication appeared in 2004 in *Knowledge Management Review*.[8] This was followed in 2005 by two articles in the *Journal of Change Management*, respectively entitled 'Connecting through communities' and 'Making the invisible visible'.[9] Others followed later. The response within the funding organisation to these publications quickly confirmed the boomerang marketing effect: a number of managers who saw that the communities-of-influence work had earned external acknowledgement and credibility became curious to learn more about it.

### Narrative writing as a journey

The narrative writing did not follow a fixed plan. Rather, it evolved to respond to what was happening in the communities. However, looking back on our tracking of the GP Advisors and other groups, it is possible to see a pattern emerging over time.

- *A history:* We often started with a history of the group, initially for members' consumption only (one group called this the 'inside story').
- *Personal portraits:* We usually created portraits of one or two selected members of the group to help people unfamiliar with communities of influence understand what kind of creatures inhabited them.
- *Discussion papers:* Sometimes we drafted papers about some theme that emerged as important.
- *Achievements log:* For some groups we established a tabular log to make the tangible results of the community's work visible (this helped secure continued funding).
- *Timelines:* We also started to construct 1-page or 2-page overviews of relevant events, forming a kind of chronicle of a community's work (these provided a more visual and succinct way of laying out the story).
- *'Influencing stories':* In some cases we collected influencing stories (a compilation of vignettes about community members), in order to give specific examples of what people were doing to share learning and influence practice. We used some of these in a letter advocating continued funding of the Primary Care Cancer Lead role, sent to the chief executives of NHS primary care organisations (*see* box for an example).

**A good idea travels across England – an influencing story**

One of the communities described in this book was that of the Primary Care Cancer Leads (PCCLs – *see* Chapter 3). The following example, documented as part of our narrative tracking, shows how an effective influencing behaviour spread from one part of the country to another by virtue of the connections between members of that community.

Because PCCLs met one another regularly, they were able to spread good ideas and practices not only locally but also across the UK. For example, a group of PCCLs in the Manchester area had noted that some of their colleagues there were not having the influence they wanted, because they were not getting access to the Chief Executive of their local NHS organisation. It would be easier to get this sort of access, they reasoned, if they could point to a written strategy for cancer care in their area, so they jointly developed one. By collaborating to write a strategy, they found they were able to work out what they wanted as a group and how it all tied in with NHS policy. Various individuals then used the strategy to 'goad local primary care organisations into action', as they put it, and one used it to impress upon a local hospital that it needed to change the way it communicated diagnoses back to general practices.

The story did not end there, however. Later, at a PCCL community gathering, a cancer lead from Yorkshire heard about the Manchester group's strategy and decided to do something similar in her area. She and her local colleagues produced their own strategy document, which was used to compare how local NHS organisations were doing and press them to raise the efficiency and quality of their care.

Finally, as mentioned, we also published externally: articles in academic journals;[10] poster presentations for conferences; and a CD presentation on communities of influence.[11]

## THE SOCIAL LIFE OF THE NARRATIVE ACCOUNTS

It should be clear by now that the narrative writing was never just for its own sake. We constantly asked ourselves what was worth capturing in writing, to what purpose, and how could we share it with others. While we ourselves did learn by doing the writing, the point of sharing the drafts was always to stimulate learning in others – community members, other health professionals, the funding organisations and government policymakers. Moreover, we grasped opportunities for influence and organisational learning as they arose, rather than just doing our research and hoping that 'the report' would have an impact. People who read our drafts posed questions that prompted us to clarify certain important issues, as the three examples below illustrate.

### 1 What are the skills of the narrative writer?

When we were drafting our second article for the *Journal of Change Management* in 2005,[12] we showed it to a number of colleagues, one of whom asked 'What kind of skills does this work require?' This question proved helpful in prompting us to articulate what expertise we, as a team, had been drawing on. This may be useful to others wondering what it takes to use narrative writing as a form of evaluation.

First, we found it took an unusual kind of writer. They needed to be able to: (i) draw on appropriate theoretical and methodological underpinning; (ii) track informal conversations and connections that do not normally get written about; (iii) create readable narrative accounts that provide specific examples and telling detail; and (iv) continually think about how the accounts will be used to stimulate reflection and learning, rather than writing them for their own sake.

We also found that the writer benefited enormously from working with colleagues from the funding organisation who could: (i) point to particular activities or groups that were worth making visible; (ii) keep an ear open for important stories and share these with the writer; and (iii) maintain the focus of the whole team on what the work was contributing more widely, especially to patients.

### 2 Are the narrative accounts any more than a subjective view?

We were also asked: 'What controls can one introduce to make sure the narrative papers are not just subjective accounts?' In our response, we explained that we saw our approach as collaborative and therefore *inter-subjective*, i.e. not the subjective account of one individual.

We find inter-subjectivity a useful term because it helps to avoid polarising between 'objective' and 'subjective'. According to Wikipedia, it is a term 'used in philosophy, psychology and sociology to describe a condition somewhere between subjectivity and objectivity, one in which a phenomenon is personally experienced (subjectively) but by more than one subject'. It acknowledges that meaning comes about through dialogue. To some extent, narrative is always inter-subjective, in that it always involves a teller, a tale, and a listener or reader – as author Richard Kearney put it, it is a 'quintessentially communicative act'.[13]

While each of our narrative accounts was largely the work of one lead author, a number of features made the writing more inter-subjective: (i) we often included multiple perspectives in the accounts; (ii) we always discussed drafts with the Macmillan team, and they were then modified to reflect those discussions; (iii) we actively shared drafts with members of the groups described (often including them as a topic for discussion at community meetings) and revised them again to reflect the responses; and (iv) we shared the narrative accounts with others – colleagues, policymakers, senior managers, etc. – to see what could be learned from their reactions, or what further influencing activity might be possible.

But perhaps the question remains: 'How do we know if a narrative account drafted by one individual is reliable?' One test of a narrative account is whether it resonates with people who took part in the events described. If this is the case, it is likely to mean it has 'veracity'. We find this term more fitting than words like 'validity', which stem from the positivist research tradition. After all, we were using the narrative writing to make the invisible visible and to stimulate reflection and learning, not to establish 'the truth'.

### 3 Isn't it 'writing by committee'?

More recently, we showed an early draft of this book chapter to a social scientist who shared our interest in language, writing and history. He wrote in an email:

> *It makes good sense that you expose your texts to comment and revision. But it is well known that good writing always comes from one author, since the quality of the language emerges not from compromise and consensus but from the individual's mastery of language. How do you deal with this?*

It was particularly refreshing to get this question from somebody who had been completely uninvolved in our work, and it prompted us to reflect more deeply on the role of the author in our narrative tracking. We realised that we had not yet clearly stated that we always had one 'lead author' for each narrative paper, and it was that person who wove together the different perspectives and stories into a coherent account. We think this both made the writing more readable and avoided the risk of 'writing by committee'.

## DISCIPLINED INFORMALITY: OUR METHODS EXPLAINED

We mentioned earlier that it was especially important in a healthcare context to be able to articulate some kind of academic or theoretical underpinning for our work. The methods we developed were informed for the main part by literature on: (i) communities of practice;[14] and (ii) complexity and emergence.[15] It was the latter that most influenced our writing, so we have tried to indicate below some of the principles we were implicitly guided by. Though these were not written down or formally agreed, we drew on our experience and research in both fields.

### Reflecting complex causality

Inspired by complexity thinking and our own experience, a fundamental premise underlying our work was that learning and influence emerge from interactions among a diverse group of human beings. It followed, in our view, that interactions were worth encouraging, noticing and tracking.

Complexity theory was developed at a time when it became technically possible to show through computer simulations that interactions among agents over time produced patterns. This phenomenon was called 'self-organisation' – patterns emerged without the need for any blueprint or architect (apart from the computer programmer who introduced the agents and the rules for their interaction).[16]

In the human realm, complexity thinking suggests that learning and innovation can emerge when diverse experiences and points of view come together and get heard. Let's look more closely at a few principles associated with 'emergence' and 'self-organisation'.

- *Connectivity*: For new insights to emerge, there needs to be just enough connectivity between people – neither too much (this can feel chaotic) nor too little (this can lead to stuck patterns of behaviour). The potential for learning and influence lies in connections.[17]
- *Diversity and disturbance*: A new point of view or a new story can disturb patterns and produce novelty. In human terms, we might describe this as change, learning or innovation.
- *Patterning*: The patterning that emerges from interaction is in constant movement. However, a pattern can become stuck (occurring over and over again). In human affairs, we can see conversations following predictable and sometimes stuck patterns. These can emerge when people are too anxious to experiment. Another factor in the human context is the ubiquitous presence of power (understood as the way in which people feel constrained in what they say for fear of damaging relationships).[18]
- *Amplification*: Causality is non-linear, meaning that small beginnings may be amplified, or they can just peter out. When a small shift of understanding occurs in one specific conversation, it may then be amplified as it gets picked up by other people and then spread through a chain of subsequent

**Amplification at work in conversations: an example**

One small example occurred in a meeting of one of the Macmillan-sponsored patient and carer groups. People were asked if they could give any examples of men using a document the group had helped to create. A male member of the group said rather pensively 'I've never thought about it this way'. A few seconds later, a woman said 'Maybe we should give it to some of the men in our partnership groups'. Another woman said 'I'd like to send it out to our prostate cancer group'. Spontaneously, the women in the group seemed to realise that they might actively talk to some of the men in their local web of contacts. Thus, the theme (of what men could gain from using the document) unexpectedly became amplified and generated new ideas and intentions.

conversations. We never know in advance which changes will be amplified and which will die out (*see* box for an example of amplification in a conversation).

### Complexity pointers for the narrative writer

How did complexity thinking guide our narrative writing? Stories are particularly congruent with complexity thinking, since they make it possible to create a context-rich account of lived experience, a way of making sense of organisational life.

> *[N]arrative can provide a different, and valuable, form of knowledge that enables researchers to engage with the lived realities of organisational life – the 'truth' that people at work live through every day. This is not a knowledge that aspires to certainty and control but rather emerges from a reflection on the messy realities of organisational practice. (Rhodes and Brown)*[19]

### Stories as fundamental to human thinking and learning

More fundamentally, as a form of expression stories are clearly central to learning and education. Indeed, research has demonstrated that we learn to tell stories from a very early age.

> *[S]torytelling is one of the first uses of language, a gradually mastered skill that is first developed in the third year and continues to develop gradually in sophistication. . . . By age ten, children have mastered the ability to tell causally well-formed stories. (Donald Polkinghorne)*[20]

Research has also shown that oral societies use(d) narrative to recall events and to find their way around without maps.[21] Even in literate societies, most people continue to experience the events in their life as connected and occurring over time. We dream in stories, we consume stories in the form of films and novels, and we tell each other about our experiences every day at work, at home and elsewhere.

Furthermore, in using the term 'narrative', we are drawing on a rich tradition. In the health sector, narrative writing has strong proponents.[22] Scholars from many other disciplines also make use of storytelling, e.g. Geertz in anthropology,[23] Van Maanen in ethnography,[24] EH Carr and later Richard Evans in history,[25] Weick in sensemaking,[26] and of course narrative research itself.[27] We have drawn considerable inspiration from all these fields. One author put it in a nutshell:

> *[D]isciplines in the social sciences ranging from sociology to ethnography and to organization studies [have] long been founded on the ability to tell a good story.*[28]

### Two modes of thinking

Many authors have advocated distinguishing two basic modes of thinking: narrative and generalisation.[29] Generalised forms of expression include opinions, general principles, theories, plans, analyses, classifications, how-to instructions and bullet-point lists, all of which are widespread in organisational life today. Many management writers and academics use generalisation and classification as a way of understanding and describing complex phenomena – they identify x types of leadership, or y kinds of teams. Ironically, even authors who write about narrative often come up with a taxonomy of stories! We think the distinction between narrative and generalised forms of expression is useful, even though in practice, people tend to blend stories and generalisations in both writing and speaking.

Generalised and analytical forms of writing have their place, but in working with communities of influence we became convinced that stories (case studies) were the best way of revealing the work for readers who had not been part of the conversations. Furthermore, we aimed to give readers enough detail to illuminate what people in the communities of influence were actually doing – and to demonstrate the nature of influence as a product of specific human interactions. This often meant actively encouraging community members to share specific examples.

Many authors point out that two fundamental features of both narrative and story are time and change. Bearing this in mind, our working definition of narrative was 'a process of connecting specific past, present or even future events in order to make sense of them'.

### Reflecting complex causality in the narrative accounts

Finally, in order to reflect our understanding of complexity and emergence, we were very careful in making any causal connections and always tried to acknowledge multiple influences. For example, we did the following:

- Included sufficient history and context to facilitate understanding and learning, paying particular attention to interactions and relationships.
- Used language that was sympathetic with this way of thinking. Terms like 'ripple effects', 'influence' and 'emerge' felt more fitting than the taken-for-granted managerial language of cause and effect, goals and targets, sender–receiver, inputs and outputs, and feedback (many of which are inherited from systems and communication theories). Metaphor and nuance mattered to us.

Avoiding simplistic causality did not mean, however, denying causality entirely. Indeed, for a written narrative to work, the connections made by the author have to seem plausible and reasonable, though not necessarily 'law-like'.

*In a narrative reconstruction one can understand that it is reasonable that things have happened the way they did: given the circumstances, one can see why the events occurred. (Donald Polkinghorne)*[30]

### Comparing our approach with other evaluation methods

Narrative methods are not unknown in evaluation. In a recent review of the field, McClintock gave several reasons why they are helpful. For example, stories 'can be used to focus on particular interventions while also reflecting on the array of contextual factors that influence outcomes'. Among three types of narrative method considered by McClintock, the one bearing the closest resemblance to ours is qualitative case studies. All the methods reviewed echoed one of our central principles, namely a focus on 'formative evaluation', meaning that they sought to 'improve the programme under study during its evaluation', as opposed to 'summative evaluation' which is more about reporting and concluding.[31]

One last comparison worth making is with evaluation of training programmes. A classic book on this topic by Kirkpatrick and Kirkpatrick[32] (first published in 1959 and still in print) makes use of a four-level model, whose elements are (in our words): (i) Reaction: did people like the learning process/event itself? (ii) Learning: did people's skills/knowledge change as a result of the educational intervention? (iii) Behaviour: did they put the skills and knowledge to use in the workplace? and (iv) Results: what was the ultimate impact of the learning? By using narrative methods, we collected evidence about all these levels. However we did not follow a step-by-step, analytical process, choosing instead to engage directly with community members and listen out for instructive stories of collaboration and influence.

## POINTS TO CONSIDER WHEN TRACKING A COMMUNITY OF INFLUENCE

Large amounts of money are spent on evaluating public services. For those interested in exploring the merits of narrative-based evaluation and the resources needed to do it, below we highlight some questions and points worth considering.

### Why do it?

Perhaps the first question to ask is 'Why do it?'. What invisible group activities are worth making more visible? This question might be followed by 'Does continued funding depend on it?'. If the answer to the last question is 'yes', it is worth probing further into whether the funding organisation (or at least someone within it) is looking for 'evaluation for learning'? In other words, is the work not just about documenting what has been done, but also stimulating learning and improvement?

### Getting off to a good start

We have found it helpful for the writer(s) to follow a community's evolution over time, ideally from the first days of its life. It is also worth ensuring that the writer is part of a team – there were five in our team, two of whom did the writing, but everybody shared relevant stories they gathered while engaging with community members. We also found it worked best for us to agree a lead writer for each narrative account, with other team members being willing to test-read early drafts as well as contributing examples and thinking.

### Distinguishing narrative from generalised forms of expression

As explained earlier, an important distinction for us was between (i) stories and examples on the one hand (narrative); and (ii) generalised statements and prescriptions on the other. Both have a place and we found it necessary to draw specific examples from people and weave them into the accounts.

### Trusting history

In organisational life, there is often pressure to come up with principles and predictions before past experience has been properly explored and made sense of. We found we had to keep our faith in the power of the retrospective account to stimulate thinking and to point the way forward. As mentioned earlier, for us narrative is a process of connecting events in order to make sense of them. It enables people to make sense of what has happened, not to predict the future.

> *[I]ts approach is different from the approach of formal science, which is primarily interested in explanation and the prediction of future events. (Donald Polkinghorne)*[33]

### A good story and a big number

There were moments when we realised how important it was to have 'a good story and a big number', especially when seeking to influence policymakers and senior managers. For example, as we tracked the life of the research group described in Chapter 5, we found it helpful to create an 'achievements log' with some striking statistics – number of papers published, tools developed, grants secured, degrees completed, chairs awarded, and so on. Nevertheless, we never abandoned narrative entirely in favour of statistics. As Etienne Wenger (author of *Communities of Practice*) has written:

> *You can tell how many marriages end in divorce, but that tells you little about the story of any given marriage.*[34]

### Employing different forms of writing over time

As mentioned, at each stage of a community's life, we thought about what form of narrative account would be most useful, e.g. 'inside stories', individual portraits, multiperspective narratives, logs of community achievements, and so on. Sometimes, especially when we were just starting to track a community, we would produce a collection of detailed raw narrative material, which could be drawn on later to construct a more streamlined account for a particular readership, e.g. senior managers responsible for funding the work. (Tongue-in-cheek, we came to refer to the most detailed narrative accounts as 'kitchen sink documents', because they seemed to contain nearly everything but the kitchen sink.)

### Judging the amount of detail needed for each group of readers

Detail matters in narrative writing, but the challenge is finding the right amount. A storyteller who provided a completely comprehensive account would 'rapidly grow maddening', as Alain de Botton beautifully demonstrated in his essay 'On Anticipation'.[35] Or, as we heard historian Simon Schama say on the radio: 'Comprehensive coverage is the enemy of storytelling'.[36] Yet too little detail and the narrative loses its richness and ability to stimulate learning.

### Choosing words carefully

In the writing, it mattered to us which words we used. Overused terms like 'input', 'feedback' or 'change management', to name just three, often carry unconscious assumptions and taken-for-granted ways of thinking. It is well worth searching for fresh language that more accurately or evocatively describes the richness, messiness and unpredictability of the real world.

### Making narrative accounts navigable

Any journalist knows that meaningful subheadings can help to tell a story. To be meaningful, they need to express an idea, i.e. say more than just 'introduction', 'lessons learned' or 'conclusions'. When headings are drawn together to form a contents page, this provides the reader with yet another way to navigate what may be a long narrative account. Another useful device mentioned earlier is a chronological list or timeline of key events in the story of the group or individual (this can show the story at a glance).

### Visual forms of communication

Mindful of the power of a picture to replace a thousand words, we gave careful consideration to which visual forms to make use of in our narrative tracking work. From the start of our work, we took photographs of people in the communities and integrated these into our internal narrative accounts, to add life and give shape to what may otherwise seem amorphous.

In general, we were economical in our use of diagrams, since these almost inevitably simplify and idealise the complexity of real life (that is of course their main attraction). Nevertheless, there were certain moments when diagrams proved useful, and complemented the writing – for example, in presenting the evolution of all the communities we had worked with over time, or in showing how many patients a relatively small professional community could potentially benefit.

In future, audio and video formats will no doubt become increasingly important, since communities can be given portable cameras, and short videos can easily be shared. Audio and video can certainly move people, but in our experience text is still invaluable for the record it secures, its potential for resurrection and its relative sophistication.

## Confidentiality

As any professional researcher knows, it is important to have ways of anticipating and responding to questions about confidentiality and anonymity. With one-to-one interviews in particular, it is crucial to check what people are willing to share with whom, so that you know what you can and can't reveal later on, say in a group meeting.

Recording is invaluable, especially if the intention is to use real spoken words in written accounts. It also enables the writer to participate fully in conversations without having to scribble all the time. Clearly, though, it is important to explain how the recording is going to be used.

One can never anticipate every concern, so it is important to be willing to respond to worries as they arise. Indeed, in our case, it sometimes became necessary to explore more than once with people 'why are we writing about this group, and how are we going to use the narrative accounts?'

In narrative inquiry, the notion of 'informed consent', commonly applied in empirical research, is not entirely appropriate. In their useful book on the subject, Clandinin and Connelly point out that narrative inquirers are doing something different from empirical research, which typically views participants 'as subjects in need of protection in research undertakings'.[37] They suggest the term 'relational responsibility' as a useful way of thinking about research ethics. This seemed precisely the right principle for our narrative tracking work, in which we viewed the people we met and talked to as participants and colleagues rather than as subjects.

Finally, it is worth being aware that narrative inquiry is risky for all the people involved – those who are written about may feel edgy about having a light shone on their story, but the writer may also feel clumsy or awkward at times. This is normal.

### Introducing narrative accounts to readers

As mentioned, we always sought to use our written accounts to stimulate learning and influence. To this end, we found that it helped if we took care to introduce the writing to our readers, e.g. through a carefully worded email, indicating what kind of response we were inviting at any particular point in time. However, despite carefully worded introductions, there may always be some people who automatically view writing as simply the product of the author, not as a group learning process. As we saw in this chapter, one way of making sure community members do engage with a narrative account is to let them know that it is about to go to external readers, especially if they are viewed as politically significant.

Another effective method we tried more recently was to pick a particularly telling, short passage from a narrative account, e.g. a real example of informal influencing in everyday working life. We then read it out loud and explored it in a community meeting. The face-to-face setting made a lively and stimulating exchange possible. Immediately afterwards (in a break) a number of people spontaneously articulated insights it had sparked for them, and the person whose story had been read out felt that it enabled the group to recognise her influencing skills.

### Beware of creating a database of stories

Once people see the value of stories, there is often a temptation to create some kind of 'story bank' (usually on a website) for people to access when they feel like it. It is advisable to test such an idea on a small scale before investing much money in it, in order to find out if people really will use it. Putting stories into a database may just serve to put them to sleep. Besides, truth does not lie in the stories themselves – learning and knowledge emerge between people as they tell, listen and respond to each other's stories, especially if the timing is right. When someone relates real experiences, often their story sparks other people to tell theirs. Hearing other people's stories generates associations and connections and can change thinking and behaviour.

## NOTES

1 See also our earlier account: Donaldson A, Lank E, Maher J. Making the invisible visible: how a voluntary organization is learning from its work with groups and communities. *Journal of Change Management*. 2005; 5(2): 191–206.

2 Boden D. *The Business of Talk: organizations in action*. Cambridge: Polity Press; 1994. pp. 8–10. See also Stacey R. *Strategic Management and Organisational Dynamics: the challenge of complexity*. 5th ed. Harlow, Essex: Prentice Hall; 2007.

3 Shaw P. *Changing Conversations in Organizations: a complexity approach to change*. London and New York: Routledge; 2002. p. 10.

4 Boden, op. cit. pp. 8–10.

5 Shotter J. The social construction of our 'inner lives'. *Journal of Constructivist Psychology.* 1997; **10**: 7–24. Available at: www.taosinstitute.net/Websites/taos/Images/Resources Manuscripts/SC_inner_lives.pdf or www.massey.ac.nz/~alock/virtual/inner.htm (accessed 23 February 2011). See also: Shotter J. *Conversational Realities Revisited: life, language, body and world.* Ohio: Taos Institute; 2008.

6 See, for example, Czarniawska B. *A Narrative Approach to Organization Studies.* London: SAGE Publications; 1998. Denning S. *The Springboard: how storytelling ignites action in knowledge-era organizations.* Boston: Butterworth-Heinemann; 2001. Gabriel Y. *Storytelling in Organizations: facts, fictions and fantasies.* Oxford: Oxford University Press; 2000. Snowden D. Narrative patterns: the perils and possibilities of using story in organizations. *Knowledge Management.* 2001; **4**(10). Also available at: www.cognitive-edge.com/articlesbydavesnowden.php (accessed 23 February 2011).

7 Personal communication with Leif Edvinsson.

8 Donaldson A, Lank E, Maher J. Using CoPs to innovate KM at Macmillan: sharing knowledge through CoPs at Macmillan Cancer Relief. *Knowledge Management Review.* 2004; **7**(5): 12–15.

9 Donaldson, *et al.* 2005; op. cit. ('Connecting through Communities', and 'Making the Invisible Visible').

10 For example: Donaldson A, Lank E, Maher J. Connecting through Communities: how a voluntary organisation is influencing healthcare policy and practice. *Journal of Change Management.* 2005; **5**(1): 71–86.

11 Donaldson A, Lank E, Maher J. *Stimulating Organizational Learning Through Networks and Communities.* Henry Stewart talk on CD; 2006. Available at: http://hstalks.com/ (accessed 23 February 2011).

12 Donaldson, *et al.* Making the invisible visible. *Journal of Change Management.* 2005; **5**(2): 191–206.

13 Kearney R. *On Stories: thinking in action.* London and New York: Routledge; 2002. p. 5.

14 Lave J, Wenger E. *Situated Learning: legitimate peripheral participation.* New York: Cambridge University Press; 1991. Wenger E. *Communities of Practice: learning, meaning and identity.* Cambridge: Cambridge University Press; 1998. Wenger E, McDermott R, Snyder W. *Cultivating Communities of Practice: a guide to managing knowledge.* Boston, MA: Harvard Business School Press; 2002.

15 Stacey 2007, op. cit. Shaw, op. cit. See also: Waldrop MM. *Complexity: the emerging science at the edge of order and chaos.* London: Penguin Books; 1992. Stacey R. *Experiencing Emergence in Organisations: local interaction and the emergence of global pattern.* London: Routledge; 2005.

16 The Santa Fe Institute, founded in New Mexico in the mid 1980s, was a particular hotbed of complexity thinking, which drew in scholars from both natural and social sciences. See Waldrop, op. cit. for a very readable account.

17 Waldrop, op. cit. p. 291.

18 For an exploration of anxiety and power in organisational life, see Stacey 2007, op. cit. and Shaw, op. cit. Stacey and Shaw draw particularly on the works of Norbert Elias, e.g. Elias N. *What is Sociology?* London: Hutchinson; 1978.

19 Rhodes and Brown, op. cit. citing Czarniawska.

20 Ibid. p. 113, citing Susan Kemper's review of research on narrative development in children.

21 Abram D. *The Spell of the Sensuous.* New York: Vintage Books; 1996. Chatwin B. *The Songlines.* London: Vintage; 1998.

22 For example, Professor Trish Greenalgh has published numerous articles on the use of narrative in health improvement research: http://myprofile.cos.com/P243302GRa (accessed 23 February 2011). See also Launer J. *Narrative-based Primary Care: a practical guide.* Oxford: Radcliffe Medical Press; 2002.

23 Geertz C. *Works and Lives: the anthropologist as author.* Cambridge: Polity Press; 1988.

24 Van Maanen J. *Tales of the Field: on writing ethnography.* Chicago: University of Chicago Press; 1988.

25 Carr EH. *What is history.* London: Penguin Books; 1990 (first published 1961). Evans RJ. *In Defence of History.* London: Granta Publications; 1997.

26 Weick K. *Sensemaking in organizations.* London: SAGE Publications; 1995.

27 For an overview, see: Rhodes C, Brown AD. Narrative, organizations and research. *International Journal of Management Reviews.* 7(3): pp. 167–88; 2005.

28 Rhodes and Brown, op. cit. p. 169, quoting Clegg 1993.

29 Bruner J. *Actual Minds, Possible Worlds.* Cambridge, MA and London: Harvard University Press; 1986. Bruner uses the term 'paradigmatic' to refer to generalised statements. See also: Czarniawska, op. cit., Kearney, op. cit., Polkinghorne, op. cit.

30 Polkinghorne DE. *Narrative Knowing and the Human Sciences.* New York: State University of New York Press; 1988. p. 117.

31 McClintock. Using narrative methods to link program evaluation and organization development. *The Evaluation Exchange.* 2003/4; **IX**(4).

32 Kirkpatrick DL, Kirkpatrick J. *Evaluating Training Programs: the four levels.* San Francisco, CA: Berrett-Koehler; 2006.

33 Polkinghorne, op. cit. p. 116.

34 Wenger, op. cit. p. 131.

35 Ibid. p. 15.

36 Simon Schama interviewed by Michael Parkinson, BBC Radio 2, 10 Nov 2002.

37 Clandinin DJ, Connelly FM. *Narrative Inquiry: experience and story in qualitative research.* San Francisco: Jossey-Bass; 2000. pp. 172–3.

## CHAPTER 3

# Working with and through doctors

### How a community of GPs made a difference to patient care

## OVERVIEW

*Taking the Macmillan GP community as a case study, we show how the 'collective voice' it developed made it easier for health professionals to advocate changes in policy and practice in the NHS. One of the early, relatively tangible service developments associated with the Macmillan GPs was the spread of systematic processes to improve care for dying patients. Another was the emergence of a further professional community that spanned the UK (the Primary Care Cancer Leads). Both these advances were helped by the efforts of a 'community within a community' – the Macmillan GP Advisors.*

*Over time, some communities grow and some shrink. At time of writing, the two larger Macmillan-sponsored professional communities had been brought together to create a 200-strong Macmillan Primary Care Community. This continues to be valued as a collective voice and source of knowledge by both the funding organisation and government policymakers, taking up a range of issues that matter to people living with cancer, including earlier detection of disease and better support for survivors.*

We rejoin the story of the Macmillan GP community in the early 2000s, at a time when the UK government was beginning to treat cancer as a priority. In 2000, it appointed a National Director for Cancer (Professor Mike Richards), set up a Cancer Services Collaborative and Cancer Action Team and published a Cancer

Plan for England.[1] Macmillan was increasingly invited to contribute to UK-wide thinking on cancer care, and this provided an unprecedented opportunity for the Macmillan GP community to influence the national cancer agenda.

As mentioned in Chapter 1, our first narrative account about the Macmillan-sponsored communities focused on the GP Advisor group. By 1999, the two existing GPAs could no longer support and coordinate the Macmillan GP community, which they themselves had helped to expand. Three further GPA appointments were therefore made and in the period 2000–05 there was a 'national group' of five GPAs. It acted as a kind of 'community within a community', working closely with Macmillan. It helped to distil the learning and ideas from the wider GP population, maintain momentum between the twice-yearly GP community meetings and strengthen links with policymakers.

The phrase 'distilling-and-connecting group' soon emerged to describe the expanded GPA group. The GPAs' continuing clinical status meant they remained 'one of us' as far as the wider GP community was concerned – so they were not seen as some distant specialist or manager who didn't understand the real, everyday challenges of general practice. Like the ordinary Macmillan GPs introduced in Chapter 1, the GP Advisors were given protected time for their influencing work. However, it had become clear that, for selected members of a community of influence, working directly with the sponsoring organisation was a task in its own right, so the GPAs were funded for two days a week rather than just one, enabling them to take on this wide-ranging role. The GPA role had a number of facets (*see* box).

### GPA roles at a glance

*Pastoral:* The GPAs looked after the Macmillan GPs (GP Facilitators) in their 'patch', which typically meant working with Macmillan local teams to identify and recruit GPs, provide induction, and then support them while they were Macmillan-funded and often beyond.

*Local influencers:* The GPAs became 'the cancer GP' in their region – they worked closely with local Macmillan teams to bring intelligence about primary care issues back into the charity and thus help it push for improvements in cancer care.

*National influencers:* The GPA group also influenced UK-wide advances in patient care; for example, it helped define the PCCL role in the NHS, and went on to act as a vital link with that community of influence (more about this later in this chapter).

*Leadership:* The GPAs acted as leaders within the wider GP community, taking prominent parts during the twice-yearly Macmillan GP conferences.

*Champion of the charity's objectives:* As well as extending Macmillan's reach, the active presence of GPAs was often helpful to fundraising teams in the regions.

## TRACKING THE IMPACT OF A 'DISTILLING-AND-CONNECTING GROUP'

A 'distilling-and-connecting' group such as the GP Advisors is there to enable a broader community of influence to make a difference, so it was important to make the role and effectiveness of this 'community within a community' visible to the funding organisation. Our history of the group appeared in 2004, and the following year we were asked in addition to review the effectiveness of the GP Advisor role by interviewing a wide range of stakeholders – including doctors, people living with cancer, Macmillan regional directors and managers, and the National Cancer Directors in England and Scotland. The paper we wrote proved an important factor in making the group and its achievements more visible to the funding organisation. In particular, the inclusion of patient and carer voices clearly made a difference – for example:

> *If a GP Advisor brings together GP Facilitators in their region and mentors them, and they all go away and share their thoughts over a cup of coffee with, say, three other GPs in their practice, and then all the other GPs that they talk to, I'd call them extremely cost-effective! How many GPs are there? 30 000? And how else would we reach them? (a person living with cancer)*

Another vital testimonial came from the National Cancer Director:

> *Having a cadre of practising GPs championing cancer in primary care had not happened in a coordinated fashion before the advent of the Macmillan GPAs. . . . The importance of primary care for cancer was recognised in the Calman Hine report but it stopped short of addressing how [to strengthen it]. Its importance was also recognised in the 2000 Cancer Plan but again it was necessary to work through what needed to be done to improve primary care in relation to cancer. The GPAs were collectively helpful in developing answers here, with different GPAs championing different aspects . . . (Professor Mike Richards, National Cancer Director, England)*

It was extraordinarily important to have GP champions for cancer, Mike Richards continued, and it would have been 'a real step backwards' if Macmillan had stopped having them in place.

## TANGIBLE AND INTANGIBLE ACHIEVEMENTS OF COMMUNITIES

Since our narrative tracking of the Macmillan-sponsored communities of influence was informed by complexity thinking, inevitably we found ourselves debating how to think about 'outcomes'. We set out to identify not just the highly tangible changes associated with community work, such as new programmes of work or written products. We also wanted to make visible the kind of things emerging at the more intangible or invisible end of the spectrum – we viewed the stories and experiences shared within the communities as important outcomes in themselves. These stories had the potential to 'ripple out' and influence thinking, policy, services and practices on the ground. In other words, the sharing of problems, solutions, ideas and experiences itself stimulated learning and change. Three short influencing stories from the GP community give a flavour of what we mean (*see* box).

### GP-influencing stories

***1 Sharing good ideas at meetings of the entire Macmillan GP community***

At a Macmillan GP conference, participants were asked to write down stories of their activities as GP Facilitators. One wrote:

> *We organised a palliative care consultant to come along to one of our multidisciplinary meetings and talk about new drugs on the palliative care menu. One of the GPs present clearly had very poor knowledge of palliative care (as those of us who had covered for his patients at weekends had discovered). However, he was using all the new drugs with gay abandon whenever he met with a rep. This identified for us an important area of work – work constructively with reps. We have negotiated with all the reps who market palliative care drugs in our locality, to present their products at the multidisciplinary groups, where their usefulness can be assessed more objectively, rather than doing individual visits to GPs. (Macmillan GP)*

***2 Using the collective voice of GPs and people living with cancer***

A group of cancer charities, including Macmillan, was putting together a joint proposal to the UK's Department of Health on priorities for cancer patients in coming years. The draft paper was circulated to the Macmillan GP community, and at one of the regular Macmillan GP conferences about 60 participants (including people affected by cancer) got a chance to comment on it. Their suggestions were collated and refined and, within a week of the conference, the people developing the policy document received a collective response from practising GPs and people living with cancer.

***3 Getting a foot in the door with local practices***

Not long after Cathy Burton became a Macmillan GP in south London in 2004, she found out there was some money available from the National Institute for Clinical Excellence (NICE – an independent organisation in the UK responsible for providing national guidance on promoting good health and preventing and treating ill health) to encourage general practices to get involved in breast screening. She knew the uptake of women going for breast screening in her three local London boroughs was quite low (about 55%).

Traditionally, primary care professionals were not at all involved with breast screening, explained Cathy, 'yet we know that women take notice of what their GPs say'. So she went out to talk to local practices about breast screening, and once she was there she could talk to them about local services more generally, if they were interested, including palliative care. 'Sometimes they just wanted to hear about the breast screening and what money they could get,' she recalled. Quite often she heard them say 'We don't have many patients with palliative care needs.' But, she added, 'I kept on chipping away'. Eventually she had practices saying they wanted to get involved in improving palliative care.

### Communities help to spread good practice

Such examples of influencing were important but we also wanted to establish whether and in what way the Macmillan GP community could be associated with some more large-scale, prominent outcomes. For example, most people agreed that the activities of the five GP Advisors and the wider Macmillan GP community helped to spread a systematic approach to caring for dying patients that had been created by Dr (later Professor) Keri Thomas, a Macmillan GP from 1998 to 2005.

Each person we spoke to told a slightly different story about the GSF, so it posed a particularly interesting challenge for the narrative writing. What people seemed to agree on was that the first seeds appeared in the late 1990s when GPs, many of whom were members of the Macmillan GP community, collectively identified an 'out-of-hours' problem – some cancer patients were being moved into hospitals or hospices during periods when the general practice surgery was closed, despite the patients' wishes to remain at home as long as possible. The Macmillan GP community highlighted the need for some practical guidelines for health professionals to ensure that patients' wishes regarding their care were respected, day or night. Two Macmillan GPs were asked to put together a report on the subject, which they did with the help of Macmillan staff. The Macmillan out-of-hours report eventually appeared in 2001, authored by Keri Thomas.[2]

### Improving care for the dying

Building on the out-of-hours work, Keri created the GSF for community palliative care. Initially intended for use by general practices and later extended to residential care homes, the GSF was a comprehensive 'toolkit' for general practices – for example, it encouraged them to keep a register of people diagnosed with cancer and to hold regular meetings to plan their care. The intention was both to improve the patient's experience and boost staff morale.

Keri played the pivotal role in piloting the GSF locally (in Yorkshire).[3] She was a good example of a practising GP who spent a number of years as part of the

Macmillan GP community and ultimately moved on to take up a position as a national clinical leader – she was appointed national clinical lead for the NHS's end-of-life care programme, launched in 2004, and also went on to work with colleagues, particularly at the University of Birmingham, to extend use of the GSF to care homes.[4]

The spread of GSF across the UK became central to the work of the wider Macmillan GP community. While the framework was being piloted by Keri in 2001, Macmillan manager Glyn Purland (the organisational sponsor for the GP community) was making the case for Macmillan to fund its spread to 1000 general practices in England during 2003–04. In the event, the 'Macmillan GSF Programme' over-achieved this target, with nearly 1500 practices adopting the processes by the end of the period, meaning that it was in use in every cancer network in England. From 2005 the spread programme was taken over by the NHS. A brief story from one of the Macmillan GPs gives an idea of what the GP community did to help spread the GSF (*see* box).

**When face-to-face meetings make a difference**

When Julian Fester became a Macmillan GP in 2003, one of the first things he did was to introduce himself to the six Macmillan nurses in his area and speak to them about the GSF. He also wrote to all local practices, and when only a few showed interest in the GSF, he went back to the Macmillan nurses to find out what the problem was. It was only in speaking to them directly that he realised he had assumed they were familiar with the GSF. In reality, they could not say exactly what it was, let alone 'sell it' to a GP. He went on to spend a morning explaining the GSF to the nurses and, at the end of it, they were 'even more fired up about it' than he was. In the next few days, practices began to contact him with enquiries about it. And when visiting one general practice, Julian heard people proclaiming the benefits of the GSF – they said patients were getting excellent care and GPs had become more supportive of one another. For example, one GP who had had difficult experiences with two dying patients now felt that, thanks to the regular meetings in his practice to discuss their dying patients, he had a team to support him.

### 'Knowledge products' created by communities

Another type of tangible outcome that often emerges from community work is a set of guidelines that members pull together offering practical advice on a particular topic for their peers. Sometimes we refer to these as 'knowledge products'. Not only are such products useful to professional practitioners and/or members of the public; they also enable community members to experience a sense of a worthwhile collective achievement.

A big advantage of GPs developing guidelines for general practices was that GPs knew how GPs worked (similar to patients creating information for patients). This meant that the material created was more likely to be used than something produced centrally by managers. It therefore had a chance of becoming a consistent part of everyday practice. Examples included: (i) a desktop blotter created by Macmillan GPs in Scotland, summarising all the relevant guidelines for cancer care; (ii) top tips compiled on a range of subjects (e.g. 'Ten top tips for palliative care'); and (iii) content for GP information systems.

Macmillan GPs were also sometimes pulled in to help create NHS guidelines. For example, Ivan Cox, who had been one of the first Macmillan GPs back in the 1990s, chaired the first group that wrote guidelines on cancer referral for GPs, published by the UK's National Institute for Clinical Excellence in 2005.

One important consideration, when a community of influence has created a set of guidelines, is to encourage them to think about giving it a 'social life'. In brief, this means giving thought to the many different ways they could encourage people to *use* the information, rather than just feeling satisfied with the product and letting it disappear into a black hole. We think these lessons about 'bottom-up' creation and dissemination are so important that we have devoted a chapter to the 'social life of documents' (*see* Chapter 4).

## A COMMUNITY OF LEADERS IN PRIMARY CARE

Another major accomplishment of the GP Advisor group was to help the NHS define and develop the new role of Primary Care Cancer Lead. Conversations among Macmillan GPs and policymakers had led to a number of initiatives springing up around the UK to develop clinical leaders who could move cancer up the healthcare agenda. A breakthrough occurred in 2000, when the Cancer Plan for England pledged £3 million a year to support a PCCL within every local NHS organisation (known at the time in England as a primary care trust or PCT), to be funded by the UK Department of Health.

The story of how this happened is a good example of how major changes emerge from very specific, local interactions (one of the fundamental premises of this book). One day Macmillan GP Advisor Ivan Cox invited National Cancer Director Mike Richards to a workshop, during which the latter apparently became convinced of the need for the Cancer Lead role. Mike Richards then invited members of the GP Advisor group to his office to work out a plan. Because the idea was distilled from GP experience, there was relatively quick agreement about how it should work.

One of the Macmillan GPAs then took on the task of defining the role more precisely, making use of the GPA group's collective influence and experience. He always put his draft papers to the Macmillan GP Advisor group for comment and adapted them in the light of the group's suggestions. He found that to say 'the GP Advisor group agrees x' is much more powerful than saying 'I think x'.

The Cancer Leads eventually appointed were about 75% GPs and 25% nurses and other professionals. They continued to work in the National Health Service, but (like the Macmillan GPs) were given 'protected time' (typically one day a week, paid for by the NHS) to look for ways to improve cancer services in the community. They typically did this by working with NHS commissioners and bringing a primary care perspective into decision-making.

Compared to the Macmillan GPs, who were chiefly concerned with peer-to-peer education and end-of-life care, the PCCL role was on the whole a more strategic one, looking at the whole of the patient's 'cancer journey', including prevention and early symptoms. (In practice, the difference between PCCLs and Macmillan GPs was not always black and white. Indeed, some individuals had both types of post, so they combined both sets of interests.)

By 2005, the PCCL role was well established in England, with 240 Cancer Leads spread across the country, and they constituted another important community of influence.

### Members focus on developing key relationships

The narrative tracking of the PCCL community revealed that what PCCLs did above all was develop useful relationships with decision-makers at national, regional and local levels. They went to meetings, persuaded people to think differently, wrote letters, and did whatever it took to build credibility and influence. In the process, they became more and more skilled influencers:

> *Many of the early PCCLs began with an interest in a particular aspect of cancer, such as palliative care or nursing, and needed to learn how to lead, how to influence, and how to think outside the box. Many of those remaining today are far more clued up . . . it is around developing relationships and credibility. That's more important than anything else – it's who you know, not just what you know.* (PCCL, Yorkshire, 2006)

#### Influencing stories from the PCCL community

The stories we collected from the PCCL community give a flavour of what form their work took in practice. We heard about networking, practice visits, sharing ideas and creating collaborative groups locally.

***1 Becoming known as the 'cancer person'***

Many PCCLs became well known locally as 'the cancer person' and thus gained influence. 'Anything with "cancer" on it gets routed to us,' said one. A London PCCL described how she visited local practices to hear what concerns they had about existing cancer services, and returned to the same practices later on to show them what action had been taken: 'You spend 20 years in an area working as a GP,' she said, 'and you hardly meet any of your GP colleagues'. Yet as a PCCL she got to know up to 80% of the GPs in her patch. (PCCL, south London)

***2 Meetings that matter***

One PCCL started a spreadsheet of all the meetings he attended and letters he wrote in trying to make progress on the cancer front – he stopped recording them when they reached 200. For example, he attended the Health Authority's Cancer Strategy Forum, Cancer Clinical Forum, palliative care meetings and meetings at the RCGP, took hospital consultants out to lunch to get to know and influence them, and bid for funding from the cancer network for various projects. (PCCL, Leicestershire)

***3 Knowing one's way around the system***

Research had suggested that PCCLs who were linked to an important NHS committee in their area (the Professional Executive Committee or PEC) were more influential than those who were not. Some were members or even chairs of their local PEC; others found it more difficult to engage with the committee. What counted in such cases, as one put it, was 'knowing your way around the systems': 'If you hit a brick wall one way, it's knowing who to go to. . . . If I get nowhere with the PEC, I know exactly where to go to ask for help, or how to embarrass those who have not been as forthcoming as they could have been'. (PCCL, Oldham, 2006)

***4 Creating local collaborative groups***

Many PCCLs created 'cancer action teams' or other multidisciplinary groups in their area (involving, for example, NHS managers, patients, GPs, nurses, practice managers, out-of-hours staff, hospital representatives, cancer specialists, public health representatives, dieticians, and smoking cessation staff). Such groups succeeded in identifying and remedying gaps in care, as well as creating 'knowledge products', such as patient information leaflets or guides for general practices.

Although the PCCL role was primarily an English phenomenon, there were similar developments in the rest of the UK and below we give examples from Northern Ireland and Scotland. Each account shows the extraordinary influence that one Macmillan GP can have, but also the value of having a group of GPs working together in a particular health economy.

## STORY OF A REGIONAL COMMUNITY OF INFLUENCE

In the beginning, Northern Ireland had just one Macmillan GP: Dermott Davison was one of the first six Macmillan GP Facilitators in the UK between 1992 and 1996. In this role, he came to develop a strong reputation as 'the cancer GP' in Northern Ireland and became involved in many cancer-related activities, including the creation of a new-build Cancer Centre at the City Hospital in Belfast.

As part of his work as a GP influencer, one of Dermott Davison's greatest contributions was in the area of undergraduate education: as a Macmillan GP, he took up a part-time Macmillan-funded lectureship in the Department of General Practice at Queen's University Belfast until 2002. There he taught palliative medicine to undergraduates and also undertook some research with a colleague, looking at (i) cancer patients' place of death and (ii) educational needs in primary care.

### A 'gang of GPs'

The group story begins in 2000, when a number of Macmillan GP appointments started to be made in Northern Ireland. By the end of 2001 there were Macmillan GPs in each of four local NHS organisations (known as health boards). Their protected time was typically funded for one day a week, and when the first three-year phase came to an end, the funding of many of the posts was picked up by the NHS. By 2003, the group numbered nine GPs.

Effectively a regional community of influence, the group was ably supported by the Macmillan team in Belfast, under the leadership of the general manager of Macmillan in Northern Ireland, Heather Monteverde, who had been Northern Ireland's first specialist breast care nurse as far back as 1986. They met as a group twice a year in Northern Ireland, as well as regularly participating in the Macmillan-organised UK-wide GP conferences. As with most groups, this one evolved over time. At the beginning the Macmillan GPs were mainly focused on visiting and educating their colleagues on palliative care, but with time they got a chance to develop further as leaders and influencers.

In the early days, there was a particular need to bridge the primary–secondary care gap – secondary care wanted to engage with GPs but didn't know how. Single GPs were perceived as just representing themselves, whereas the Macmillan GPs came to be seen as a group that the local Boards and Trusts could call on. Or to put it another way, there was no longer any 'excuse' for secondary care not to talk to GPs. Heather summed it up as follows.

> *They've achieved an incredible amount. And I think the success was having nine at one time instead of dribs and drabs. . . . The point was it was a collective, not just one GP struggling alone. (Heather Monteverde)*

### GPs help create a new multidisciplinary network

Meanwhile, another important part of the cancer story in Northern Ireland was the formation of the Northern Ireland Cancer Network (NICaN). Like England, in the early 2000s, Northern Ireland was giving priority to improving cancer care. The Campbell Report ('Cancer services: investing in the future') had been published in 1996, and about two years later the chief executives of the four health boards set up the Campbell Commissioning Group to implement the report's recommendations. Macmillan GP Dermott Davison was invited to be a member of this group, which concluded in 2002 that there was no body (other than the group itself) offering a regional perspective on cancer care, and that this might lead to inequity for patients. To give just one example, information and services related to reconstructive surgery for breast cancer patients varied considerably from one area to another.

Macmillan was instrumental in the planning and shaping of NICaN, contributing more than £1 million to it in total. As a UK charity, it brought to the table its extensive experience with the English cancer networks, which were largely populated by specialists. Gradually consensus emerged that primary and palliative care should be a substantial component of NICaN's work.

The process of forming NICaN began in earnest when Heather and colleagues put together a bid to Macmillan and secured funding for four lead posts: as well as Lead GP Dermott Davison, there was a Lead Clinician, a Lead Nurse, and a Manager for the Network. Further posts were later established, using a variety of public and charitable funding sources. The posts included: an administrative officer, a patient and public involvement coordinator, a supportive and palliative care coordinator, a service improvement lead, a patient information post, and a chemotherapy manager.

Thus, by 2004 there were two interconnected groups dedicated to improving cancer care in Northern Ireland – the Macmillan GPs and NICaN. As well as being a product of collaboration between Macmillan and other decision-makers in Northern Ireland, NICaN was also a kind of community of influence in its own right. Important advances in patient care followed. For example, 'out-of-hours boxes' and handover forms for palliative care patients came to be established in every Health Board. This 'would have been unheard of' five years earlier, commented Heather Monteverde.

In a conversation with us in the Belfast Macmillan office in 2007, Heather and two of the Macmillan GPs reflected on what had made the difference. 'Relationships' and 'being at the table' seemed to be key factors. Northern Ireland is a very small place, Heather explained, where everybody knows everybody and things get done through personal relationships rather than at 'big strategic meetings where the consultants don't know each other'. The GP group was like 'a pool of knowledge' that could be tapped into as needed, to make things happen.

### Continuing influence despite upheavals in local health economy

We emphasise in this book that one of the great strengths of communities of influence is that they can survive organisational restructuring, which is a frequent occurrence in the NHS. In 2007, all the structures in the Northern Ireland health scene were in a state of flux, following a review of public administration in the region, and the health boards were to be scrapped and replaced by new structures. At the same time, there was a sense that there was still a way to go to create understanding of what primary care was capable of in terms of cancer and supportive care.

As an established group, the Macmillan GPs in Northern Ireland were in a good position to continue influencing in the new landscape. For example, they found their way into various important new groups such as local commissioning groups, strategic groups created to improve cancer and palliative care, and 'pathfinder primary care partnerships' (set up to facilitate collaboration in each locality, by bringing together GPs, social work and public health professionals, local politicians, and lay and community members). They also got involved in an initiative designed to transform follow-up care for cancer survivors in Northern Ireland.

## PORTRAIT OF A SCOTTISH INFLUENCER

The twice-yearly PCCL conferences tended to have a presence from every part of the British Isles. To give an idea of the kind of person we encountered at the PCCL community meetings, below is the story of Bob Grant, a Macmillan GP and PCCL in Scotland.

Bob's story begins in 1960 when, at the age of 14, he started to find it difficult to walk to school. He was admitted to hospital in Aberdeen, where he was treated for cancer (a non-Hodgkin's lymphoma) in his thigh bone. Bob's experiences of being an adolescent in hospital (both positive and negative) strengthened his interest in studying medicine. Later, when he checked his own records at medical school, he found that there had been 'no great expectation of survival' at the time of his cancer treatment.

In 1981, Bob settled into a two-doctor general practice in Fife, and in the early 1990s, despite persistent infections in his bad leg, he embarked on his first real influencing role as 'GP Advisor to the Fife Health Board'. He worked with a public health colleague and Macmillan to create a Lead Cancer Team in Fife. All of its members (Bob, plus a gastroenterologist, a nurse and an administrator) were in Macmillan-funded posts, and their funding was later picked up by the local NHS organisation (the Fife Health Board). Bob's role made him the first Lead GP for Cancer in the UK (in effect he was both a Macmillan GP and a Primary Care Cancer Lead) and gave him two days a week of protected time. He retained the Macmillan tag long after his charity funding ceased.

The Cancer Lead Team concept proved successful in Scotland for a number of reasons, including high-level backing, the calibre of the members and their contacts, regular meetings, office space and full-time administrative support. Five influential years followed until the political relationships and backing weakened and people moved on.

As a 'Lead GP for Cancer', Bob was an early proponent of the 'practice visit'. He wanted to find out what his peers thought about existing cancer services in the secondary sector, so he started visiting local practices. He found they were keen to cooperate, and he unearthed a good deal of information he would not have found through a paper survey. Ultimately he visited every practice in the area – about 63 in total – in just under two years, and sent his typed-up notes back to the practices, inviting their comments. After every five visits, he sent his findings to consultants from the secondary sector and also presented them to the Fife Cancer Board.

> *The collated visit reports drove the agenda of the Cancer Board, because we were picking up so many concerns. We were bringing information from practices that was unknown to the Board. This really did make a difference, and I could go back to see the GPs again afterwards to show action was being taken. For example, we learned that there were deficiencies in the urological cancer service, so we worked with the consultants and lobbied for an extra consultant in this field. (Bob Grant)*

Unfortunately, Bob's leg problems were to return. In 2001 he fell and broke his bad leg while walking his dog. It turned out to be a pathological fracture that was not going to heal, and it looked like he was going to have to stay on antibiotics indefinitely. In 2002, he looked in the mirror and didn't like what he saw, so he requested an amputation. Fortunately, the operation went well; he had no postoperative infections and was home by Christmas, walking on a false limb.

One day in 2003, as he was enjoying getting active again, Bob had the idea of raising money for Macmillan by doing the entire coastal path walk around Fife – 108 miles – on crutches. In August, he set out with his family and dog, and they were joined by groups of ramblers. Macmillan fundraisers organised press coverage and the walk succeeded in raising £16 000 for charity.

Not long after, pain returned and further investigations showed that the main artery to the stump had got blocked off as a late reaction to the radiotherapy, aggravated by wearing a false limb. So, from November 2003 Bob ceased wearing a limb and instead got about 'even faster than before' on some special crutches. By July 2004 he was ready to go back to work by joining a general practice in Fife on a part-time basis.

A few months later, Bob applied successfully for the chairmanship of the newly established Scottish Cancer Group. In his first year as chairman he learned to 'understand the system', work with the Scottish Executive (Scotland's national government) and collaborate with patient representatives. He also visited each of the five NHS cancer centres in Scotland. In this period, several advances happened – job vacancies were filled, waiting times were reduced and patient care improved.

At the end of 2005, Bob also joined a group within the UK's National Cancer Research Institute looking at cancer in teenagers and young adults. Given his personal experiences, these objectives were close to his heart. The group's aim was to organise research, identify gaps in services, and coordinate clinical trials.

Reflecting on his career, Bob emphasised the support from family and colleagues during his chronic illness, adding that Macmillan was 'absolutely crucial in Scotland in the whole development of the Cancer Lead role and in keeping the GPs together'.

It is notable how Bob's personal experience informed his role as he developed from 'ordinary GP' to 'national influencer', and also how he made good use of collaborative groups along the way (e.g. the Scottish Cancer Lead Team and the PCCL community).

## WHAT INVESTMENT IS NEEDED TO KEEP PEOPLE CONNECTED?

Working with professional communities of influence requires support and investment. For each of the two larger communities described so far, the arrangements differed slightly, reflecting different histories and the involvement of different types of people, as we show below.

### Support for the Macmillan GP community

In the case of the Macmillan GPs, the charity both funded their protected time and supported the community by putting in place:

- a rigorous selection process: the GPs were interviewed both by Macmillan local managers and by the responsible Macmillan GP Advisor, and if no suitable candidate came forward, no appointment was made
- regular face-to-face meetings for the community, with skilled community facilitation
- local and regional steering groups, typically including representatives of the local NHS organisations, as well as a palliative care specialist, a Macmillan GP Advisor, and someone from the local Macmillan team
- information and administrative help, including access to the Macmillan library, induction packs, videos, and an email group for Macmillan GPs UK-wide
- GP academic posts: a few members of the Macmillan GP community held such positions, which helped to generate much-needed evidence for improvements in care (*see* Chapter 5).

In return, Macmillan GPs were typically asked to produce an annual report describing who they had been in contact with, what kind of educational activities they had run, what stories they had heard, and how they had developed their own skills or qualifications.

### Testing the option of support without ownership: the PCCL community

In contrast with the Macmillan GPs, Macmillan chose not to go for badging or 'ownership' of the PCCLs. Instead it left the funding of protected time to the NHS and concentrated all its investment on supporting and staying connected with community members by funding a dedicated 'Macmillan Support Programme' (MSP) for them. This continued for six years (2001–06), providing the Cancer Leads with opportunities to network and develop their leadership and influencing capacities, including:

- twice-yearly conferences – to meet one another and share experiences and ideas about influencing the health service
- opportunities to go into more depth with peers in small regional groups ('learning sets'), with professional facilitation
- professional development, including induction sessions and help with personal development planning
- funding for projects – one, for example, was focused on cancer prevention awareness in schools
- access to Macmillan nurses and Macmillan regional teams – a chance to work in partnership to develop services for people living with cancer.

In other words, with the PCCL community, Macmillan was testing whether giving extensive support to members, without actually funding any protected time, was a better and more cost-effective way of developing and maintaining close links with a group of influential professionals. Evaluations showed that the PCCLs greatly appreciated the educational programme and the community gatherings; most of them were new to strategic and managerial responsibilities.

When the Macmillan Support Programme for the PCCL community came to its planned end in 2006, two years of uncertainty and turbulence followed. The NHS was under pressure to make dramatic savings and it proved hard for PCCLs, as lone voices in a hospital-driven environment, to hold on to their protected time – the cancer agenda in England was focused around the cancer networks, which were largely specialist. Not surprisingly, PCCL numbers dwindled – the community had peaked at around 240 in 2005, but by 2010 it was closer to 100. Some new PCCLs were appointed by the NHS between 2006 and 2010, but these individuals did not have the history, educational support programme or the relationships that had been built up by the earlier cohort. Above all, once the opportunities to talk as a group disappeared, momentum was lost.

Furthermore, during this period, Macmillan itself was restructuring, organisational sponsor Glyn Purland retired and community facilitator Lorraine Sloan moved into another role. It therefore became difficult for Macmillan to sustain a relationship with the PCCLs as a separate community. For a while, a drug company offered some sponsorship, enabling two further conferences to be held. However, the nature of these meetings was different. This suggested that, once a charitable sponsoring organisation withdraws support from a community of influence, others can attempt to take over the network of relationships cultivated over time, but the spirit of the community may be lost.

## CAN RELATIONSHIPS SURVIVE A LOSS OF COMMUNITY MOMENTUM?

It is worth reflecting on the challenges of maintaining relationships during such a hiatus in community support. Clearly, sponsors do not want their investment to be lost – so they may want to find ways to stay in touch with members and 'keep the learning' from the community before it evaporates or disperses.

In Macmillan's case, one way of staying in touch with the PCCLs was to offer them 'adoption'. Under this arrangement, the remaining PCCLs would become 'Macmillan professionals', which included being Macmillan-badged (like the Macmillan GPs), receiving invitations to Macmillan conferences and benefiting from education, newsletters and access to project grants. In other words, Macmillan could keep them within the Macmillan family without being responsible for their 'backfill funding' and without providing a dedicated support programme.

Some 10–20% of the PCCLs took up this offer, but for others there was either inadequate support from the local NHS organisations (upon whom they relied for their protected time) or insufficient interest from the individuals. The silver lining to this story was that, after the PCCLs stopped operating as a distinct community, a number of members did stay in touch and continued to work with Macmillan on a range of initiatives. This was an example of how a few mature relationships may continue long after the professionals stop meeting as a group.

### Continuity through a skilled community facilitator

After a period working elsewhere in Macmillan, Lorraine Sloan resumed her role as community facilitator for the GP community. Despite the interruption in her role, she held the history of the community in her memory more than anyone else.

Around the same time, the remaining PCCLs were invited to join the Macmillan GPs and form what was in effect a new community of influence – the 200-strong 'Macmillan Primary Care Community', and Macmillan replaced the twice-yearly GP meetings with an annual Primary Care Conference. Lorraine did what was needed to connect this enlarged community into Macmillan and make its work more visible within the charity – for example, the charity's events' department took over organisation of the conferences. She was greatly helped by her established relationship with many community members, especially one individual who had emerged as a clinical leader (Rosie Loftus – *see* Chapter 6).

### Using e-newsletters to keep in touch between meetings

Over the next three years, the relationship between Macmillan and its Primary Care Community became an arm's-length one compared to earlier times. Members met as a whole community only once a year, and Macmillan adopted a less intense way of keeping in touch between meetings – namely, through a new quarterly publication called *Primary Care Update*, which began to appear in 2008. This is a succinct and practical quarterly electronic newsletter for GPs managing cancer in primary care, including useful information (e.g. 'Top tips for safety netting', giving practical suggestions on how to avoid patients with cancer 'slipping through the net' and remaining undiagnosed) and links to other sources of help. It reaches a large number of GPs in the UK and is sent out to most NHS primary care organisations.

Though the relationship between community and sponsoring organisation was more arm's length than before, the expanded size of the community meant that it could potentially extend Macmillan's reach even further (*see* box).

#### How many people can 200 community members reach?

It is important for a sponsoring organisation to have an estimate, however rough, of community reach and impact. In the case of the Macmillan-sponsored Primary Care Community, community facilitator Lorraine Sloan developed the following calculation.

***General practice numbers***

A single Macmillan GP can potentially engage with up to 20 local practices, i.e. up to 80 GPs (four GPs per practice on average).

Two hundred GPs working in this way could potentially influence the behaviour of up to 16 000 GPs, representing approximately half the GPs in the UK, based on the assumption that there are over 30 000 GPs registered in the UK.

Even though this is a very rough-and-ready estimate, the *potential* of reaching half the entire population of the country does give an indication of just how far the influence of the GP community could reach. Moreover, the figures can be used to create a simple 'ripple effect' diagram, to explain to those outside the community, not least the budget holder, how a relationship with 200 active health professionals could potentially extend the organisation's reach and complement the work of its employees and other health professionals.

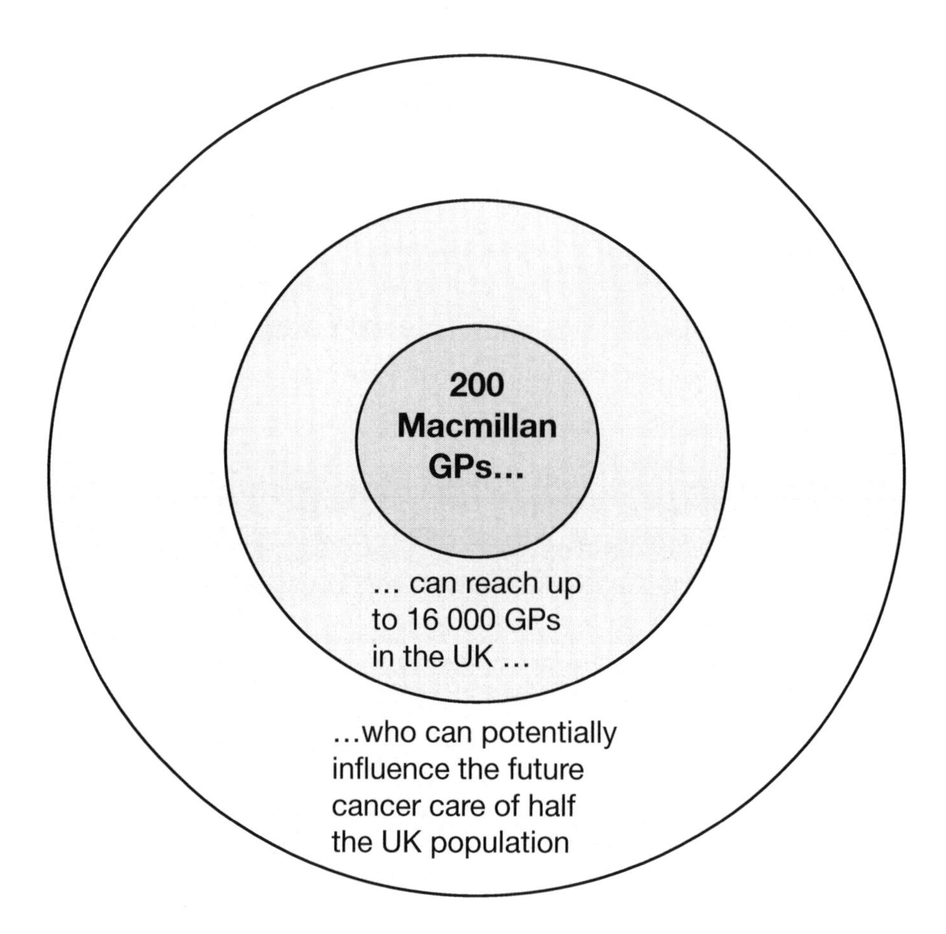


**FIGURE 3.1** Potential community reach

## FURTHER OPPORTUNITIES FOR AN ESTABLISHED COMMUNITY

At time of writing, the Macmillan Primary Care Community was continuing to influence a range of issues linked to cancer care, demonstrating the value of sustaining a community of influence over time. There is still plenty to do, based on current cancer statistics, which tell a rich story (*see* box).

**The changing story about cancer**

Cancer remains a serious and widespread illness: nearly 300 000 new cases of cancer are diagnosed each year in the UK, and more than one in three people will develop some form of cancer in their lifetime.[5] And research has shown that cancer is the number one fear for the British public, topping the list over Alzheimer's, heart attack and terrorism.[5] Better care, support, information and education are needed to improve the experience of people afraid of, or living with, cancer.

Cancer mortality rates have fallen in the UK over the last 30 years, but cancer still causes one in four of all deaths;[5] the need to support dying patients will never go away, and further work is needed to make sure people have 'a good death'. Place of death is viewed by some as an indicator of the success of services provided.[6] Studies have shown that many patients want to die at home but recent figures indicate that only about a quarter of cancer deaths in England and Wales occur at home.[7] More cancer patients could die where they wish to if more could be done to equip primary care teams to support them and their families.

The most striking fact is that the cancer story has been changing in recent years. There is now an urgent need to do more for the growing numbers of cancer survivors. Popular perception used to be that, if you got cancer, you were either cured and were perfectly well, or you died quickly of it. But survival rates have doubled in the last 40 years,[5] and better chances of survival are reflected in the size of the survivor population: 2 000 000 people in the UK today have had a cancer diagnosis, and if this number continues to rise by 3% a year, we could see 4 000 000 people living with cancer by 2030.[8] Of those who die, an increasing number will live with incurable disease for several years before their health declines irreversibly.

Of those who are cured of cancer, perhaps a quarter will experience significant problems related to treatment. The problem of 'late effects of treatment' first came to light through the determined struggle of a group of women suffering terrible side effects some 20 years after aggressive radiotherapy treatment for breast cancer during the 1970s and 1980s.[9] Although the particular set of circumstances that led to their problems may never happen again, complex cancer treatment is not risk free.

In response to this changing cancer story, in 2009 Macmillan Cancer Support and the UK government launched a National Cancer Survivorship Initiative (NCSI), which includes a project group focused on consequences of cancer and its treatment.[10] The initiative has access to the knowledge of Macmillan-sponsored communities of influence.

### Some further areas of work being pursued in 2010

A few further examples demonstrate the scope of ongoing influencing activities by the Macmillan Primary Care Community.

#### *Improving support for cancer survivors*

To help those suffering from the consequences of cancer treatment, Macmillan GPs were pressing for general practices to track what treatment cancer patients have had, so that any side effects could be picked up, even if they show themselves only years after treatment.

#### *Encouraging better care through incentive systems*

One key field of influence in recent years has been the Quality Outcomes Framework (QOF) – the annual incentive programme, introduced as part of the GP contract in 2004, which influences practice funding and GP salaries. Macmillan was the only cancer charity that made detailed submissions to the Department of Health in the first three 'QOF rounds'. In the first round (2006), Macmillan helped get QOF points established for processes designed to improve the quality of end-of-life care. Macmillan's response to the 2009 QOF consultation emphasised that its recommendations were based on extensive consultation with the Macmillan Primary Care Community.

#### *Improving the quality of GP reviews for cancer patients*

Further work has been under way to improve the quality of 'cancer reviews' by GPs. These qualify for QOF points, but there is great variation in how thoroughly they are being carried out. Macmillan can draw on the collective experience of its Primary Care Community to make a case for improving consistency in this aspect of care.

#### *Advising the UK government on cancer in primary care*

The UK government's 2010 White Paper, *Equity and Excellence: liberating the NHS*, envisaged GP consortia taking over the commissioning role in the NHS. At the 2010 Macmillan Primary Care Conference, National Cancer Director Mike Richards stated publicly that those present represented a strong community of GPs with an expertise in cancer, and he suggested that they could help recently appointed Health Minister Andrew Lansley address some of the challenges in cancer in primary care.

#### *Promoting early detection of cancer*

The Macmillan GP Advisors were involved in a stream of work led by the Department of Health aimed at improving awareness and early detection of cancer. Cancer diagnosis presents major challenges to professionals in primary care: while a few patients visiting their GP have already had cancer diagnosed, many others come into the practice with symptoms that may or may not suggest cancer as a possible diagnosis. In 2010, Mike Richards was exploring with Macmillan how the charity could support this work, drawing on its Primary Care Community as a source of knowledge as well as a network to influence behaviour on the ground.

We hope it has become clear by now that, by cultivating groups of professionals who wanted to make a difference, Macmillan continues to help improve healthcare from the ground up. This allows quality improvements to be driven by the experience and knowledge of clinicians, not by top-down government policy alone. As Lorraine Sloan summed it up: 'bottom-up influence is needed in a complex system.'

## POINTS TO CONSIDER WHEN FORMING A COMMUNITY OF PROFESSIONALS

Below we draw together some themes and insights that have emerged from our experience with the communities described in this chapter. They are intended as a starting point to stimulate thinking.

### Personal qualities needed

When we were reviewing the effectiveness of Macmillan's GP Advisor group, we took stock of the qualities that made an effective community influencer. These are probably relevant for every member of a community of influence – for example, having a passion for what they do, having credibility with peers, being a good listener and having a talent for 'herding cats'.

### Allowing flexibility for people to do what they do best and what's needed

People setting up a community of influence may be tempted to define the role of its members in advance. In practice, however, roles always vary according to current priorities as well as individuals' interests and expertise. With the GP and PCCL communities, it worked best to allow considerable flexibility in how people took up their roles – playing to the strengths of different individuals. Later on, when members have settled into their influencing role, it may be possible to specify more exactly what activities are typical.

### Choosing whether to go for 'ownership' or support

The PCCL example shows that it was possible for a funder to choose to *support* a community even when members' protected time was funded by another organisation (in this case the NHS). This is arguably a good use of charitable funds. However, there are also risks associated with such arrangements: the challenge is to find a good mix of funding (e.g. protected time, support and facilitation, or just community membership as a benefit in its own right).

### Getting funding levels right

Our review of the GP Advisor group, mentioned earlier, highlighted the importance of adequate funding levels. For example, a member of the Macmillan GP community could do their educating and influencing work with one day of protected time per week. A member of a distilling-and-connecting group may need more. Essential though it was, 'protected time' was only part of the funding. Communities of influence also needed money for meetings, travel, administrative support, and so on.

### Responding to the political context

Some of the major contributions made by the GP community emerged at times when the political climate in the UK was most favourable (the early 2000s). Later on, the environment became more challenging, so it was important to find ways to keep the momentum going (once members had left it was much harder to stay in touch) and to make the community's achievements visible to funders and decision-makers. Despite the inevitable ups and downs of this kind of work, where money and politics hold sway, one of the advantages of working through communities of influence is that, even if they shrink at times, many relationships live on. They may even resurface later on, a bit like rhizomes that work underground and re-emerge as seasons change.

### Cultivating links between community and funding organisation

We found that community members were typically more effective if they were well connected with relevant parts of the funding organisation, and if their contribution was communicated well to all stakeholders. If the funding organisation has regional teams, productive collaboration may be more likely if these are involved in recruitment of community members, negotiations around funding and objective setting. In the case of the GPA group, for example, the individuals were 'jointly owned' by Macmillan's regional offices and the four UK nations (Scotland, Wales, Northern Ireland and England), with objectives set jointly. This had the advantage of anchoring the GPAs in local health structures while also ensuring they continued to develop national connections. Furthermore, the GPA group meetings rotated around different parts of the country.

The stories told here about the GPs in Northern Ireland and Scotland also show that there are situations where it makes sense to create a regional subcommunity within a larger community of influence. The Northern Irish GPs were able to work closely with the Macmillan office in Belfast and to influence the local health economy.

### Managing entries and exits

Finally, entries and exits – how people join a community, how long they stay in it, and how they leave it – need careful thought. Inviting members to join a community is different from recruiting people for a job. For example, it is important to think about whether the invitation is to be open or whether, given the centrality of relationships to this kind of work, a degree of 'cherry picking' for the right mix of personal qualities may actually be helpful.

Regarding exits, it is worth being aware that, if members stay in a community for too long or have a personal agenda that is not in tune with the community's goals, they may get disillusioned or cynical. There is much the supporting team (*see* Chapter 6) can do to help people find the right moment to end their formal involvement and to feel 'complete' about leaving the community, thus preserving goodwill on both sides.

## NOTES

1 Department of Health. *The NHS Cancer Plan: a plan for investment, a plan for reform.* London: Department of Health – Crown Copyright; 2000. Available at: www.dh.gov.uk/en/Publicationsandstatistics/Publications/PublicationsPolicyAndGuidance/DH_4009609 (accessed 23 February 2011).

2 Thomas K. *Out-of-Hours Palliative Care in the Community.* London: Macmillan Cancer Relief; 2001. Available at: http://be.macmillan.org.uk/be/s-209-toolkits.aspx (accessed 23 February 2011).

3 Thomas K. *Caring for the Dying at Home: companions on the journey.* Oxford: Radcliffe Publishing; 2003.

4 Badger F, Shaw K, Hewison A, Clifford C, Thomas K. Gold Standards Framework in care homes and advance care planning. *Palliative Medicine.* 2010; **24**: 447–8.

5 http://info.cancerresearchuk.org/cancerstats/keyfacts/Allcancerscombined/ (accessed 23 February 2011).

6 Davies E, Linklater KM, Jack RH, *et al.* How is place of death from cancer changing and what affects it? Analysis of cancer registration and service data. *British Journal of Cancer.* 2006; **95**(5): 593–600.

7 Statistic supplied directly by Macmillan Cancer Support, based on data from Office of National Statistics.

8 www.macmillan.org.uk/GetInvolved/Campaigns/Survivorship/Livingwithorbeyondcancer.aspx (accessed 23 February 2011).

9 Hanley B, Staley K. *Yesterday's Women: the story of R.A.G.E.* London: Macmillan Cancer Support; 2006.

10 'The aim of the NCSI is, by 2012, to have taken the necessary steps to ensure that survivors get the care and support they need to lead as healthy and active a life as possible, for as long as possible. . . . The initiative is a partnership between the Department of Health and Macmillan Cancer Support and is co-chaired by the National Cancer Director, Professor Mike Richards, and the Chief Executive of Macmillan, Ciaran Devane.' www.ncsi.org.uk/ (accessed 23 February 2011).

## CHAPTER 4

# The social life of documents

## Making sure written products of communities get noticed and used

### OVERVIEW

*Many people in organisational life create perfectly good documents that end up disappearing into a black hole, and communities of influence are no exception. The creation of guidelines can be one of the more visible and valuable results of a community's work (which is why we sometimes refer to them as 'knowledge products'), but further effort is essential if these products are to have a 'social life' and influence practices on the ground.*

*Taking examples, mainly of documents created by members of the Macmillan-sponsored communities, a number of insights emerge about how to make written information influential: (i) it matters who writes a document; (ii) documents stand a better chance of influencing if they are personally introduced (ideally during a face-to-face conversation); (iii) good documents may go dormant for a while but can be revived and become influential when the time is right; and finally, (iv) look and feel also make a difference. These principles hold whether people are given a printed version, receive the document as an email attachment or obtain it from a website.*

One thing that often emerges from the conversations of a community of influence in the health sphere is the desire to document and share experience of good practice whether for fellow professionals or for patients and carers. As well as being potentially useful, this can make the community more visible and reassure funders that it is producing some tangible results. There are risks, however. Such documents may end up gathering dust and fail to influence practice; they may be treated as just more unwelcome instructions from on high, or some health professionals may follow the recommended guidelines or processes in a mechanical way. This phenomenon seemed so important that we decided to devote a chapter to exploring why it happens and what can be done about it. All of these risks can be mitigated if people are mindful of the fact that most good-practice documents are supposed to stimulate a useful conversation between patient and professional, not to be followed slavishly and act as a substitute for good communication.

## UNREAD AND UNLOVED

In healthcare, guidelines, protocols, plans, strategies, policy papers and reports come out every day. It goes almost without saying that writing can be an arduous and time-consuming process. Yet, despite the effort that goes into documents, many end up unread, unloved and rapidly forgotten. A short example may be helpful. In Chapter 1, we mentioned a report called *Breaking Bad News*. The background was that patient self-help groups had said that hospital consultants needed to get better at communicating cancer diagnoses to patients. Auditable guidelines were therefore drawn up, based (unusually at the time) on what both patients and doctors had said.

In other words, plenty of different perspectives were considered in creating the guidelines. Yet they were not implemented. So, what did happen to them? First, they were tested in two multidisciplinary teams in the UK. The reaction from the team in Hertfordshire was particularly instructive. It made clear that it would be very difficult to measure outcomes (how people felt), and that the problem was not just about the doctor–patient consultation (so not just a question of training the consultants). Procedures needed to change too, e.g. making sure that patient notes were available to consultants at least 90% of the time, and inviting GPs to see patients following diagnosis.

What this small example suggests is that, although it may be important to create guidelines, they can change behaviour only if the ground is well prepared, i.e. if people find out what needs to happen to make implementation possible. In a sense, writing down best practice is the easy part – what often prevents good guidelines from being influential is that nobody takes seriously the need to engage with the 'messy' reality of day-to-day management and clinical practice.

The silver lining to this story was that a large hospital in Hertfordshire went on to create a special 'breaking bad news clinic' (from the patients' point of view, they were simply going to a hospital appointment in the department relevant to their disease). The clinic, which was still going strong at the time of writing, drew directly on the *Breaking Bad News* guidelines. In addition, staff (consultants and nurses) underwent appropriate training and patients were given written information.

## THE VALUE OF INTERWEAVING WRITING AND TALKING

Stepping back from this specific example, one way of thinking of documents in general is that they are tools or artefacts, which stimulate learning or spread knowledge only when someone uses them. In other words, if they are to influence practice, documents need to be circulated and/or personally introduced, noticed, read, thought about, discussed and acted upon. In short, they need a 'social life', a phrase inspired by the title of Brown and Duguid's book, *The Social Life of Information.*[1] Other authors make similar points:

> *[By] writing down a law, creating a procedure, or producing a tool . . . a certain understanding is given form. This form then becomes a focus for the negotiation of meaning, as people use the law to argue a point, use the procedure to know what to do, or use the tool to perform an action . . . we discuss what we read in order to compare and enrich our interpretations. (Etienne Wenger)*[2]

> *Instead of focusing attention on the tool, the perspective I am suggesting focuses attention on how the tools are used. (Ralph Stacey)*[3]

So, why is it that many documents have a limited influence? One explanation is that most people unconsciously view communication, especially writing, as 'sending and receiving'. They circulate an email and assume it conveys the meaning intended. It easily slips their mind that, although documents may *contain useful information,* this does not automatically guarantee learning or influence. How often do people say in frustration: 'It's in the instructions' or 'Just read the report – it contains all the answers'. The danger is that, when people send out a document, they assume that they have accomplished their task, but in fact their thinking will have an influence only if people really engage with it.

A number of metaphors can be used to describe this phenomenon. We generally use 'social life', but another way of thinking about it is that, once written, a document is in a sense dead or comatose – until it is brought back to life by people, through reading and conversation. One can think of this as the need to resurrect a document that has died, or to awaken or resuscitate a piece of writing that has gone comatose. One author put it like this:

> *The deadness of the text, its removal from the living human lifeworld, its rigid visual fixity, assures its endurance and its potential for being resurrected*

> *into limitless living contexts by a potentially infinite number of living readers. (Walter J Ong)*[4]

In other words, paradoxically, it is the very deadness or 'fixity' of written documents that makes them such an excellent medium for capturing, setting out and sharing insights reached jointly by community members. Conversations are by nature transient, but writing makes it possible to preserve and share something of what people have talked about.

In the rest of this chapter, we describe a number of real examples of documents that emerged from communities of influence and how they were (or were not) given a social life. The stories bring out a number of themes: (i) the best guidelines are those created by the very kinds of people who are going to need the information; (ii) the same people can play a key role in getting 'their creation' into people's hands; (iii) if they are to make a difference, documents may need a champion (an 'introducer') who personally places them in the hands of the people they are meant to influence; (iv) good documents, even if they temporarily go into a coma, can be resuscitated when the time is right; and (v) the shape and quality of a document can strongly influence whether it is used or not. We look at each of these themes in turn below.

## BOTTOM-UP IS BEST

> *What worries me is all the money being spent on documents which are then stuffed into cupboards or boxes or don't get displayed very well at the hospital. I think* Our Principles of People-Centred Care *is an excellent example of how things* do *work. (person living with cancer, member of Macmillan patient and carer group)*

One particular written product – a document called *Our Principles of People-Centred Care* – was created by one of the Macmillan-sponsored communities of influence (a patient and carer group). The story of this publication demonstrates well how effective a combination of talk and text can be. It is worth telling in some detail, in order to show the myriad conversations that went into both creation and dissemination of this piece of writing – note that when we refer to the 'social life of documents', we are pointing to what goes on before as well as after publication.

### Created by people affected by cancer . . . with a little help

In 2003, Macmillan had brought together about 15 patients and carers to inform and contribute to its work with doctors. Another individual central to this story was

Macmillan employee Lorraine Sloan (first introduced in Chapter 2). At the time, she was community facilitator both for this group and for the Macmillan GP community. The creation of the document that came to be known as *Our Principles of People-Centred Care* was in itself a collaborative effort – many people were involved in developing the thinking that eventually crystallised in printed versions.

The story started in earnest when Lorraine, as part of her job, was asked by Macmillan to conduct a literature review to explore the meaning of 'patient-centred care' (a phrase that was central to Macmillan's work with its medical community) from the perspective of people affected by cancer. She began by identifying a number of articles, pulling out patient quotes into a large spreadsheet. She found that the quotes fell naturally under headings representing the various stages of the cancer care pathway, although mostly based around a hospital setting. It was not long before people started referring to the draft as 'the cancer journey document'. Lorraine explained to us what happened next. It is worth reproducing her words in full, because they make visible the range of conversations that helped to shape the writing:

> *With the help of Jane Bradburn (Macmillan's user involvement advisor at the time), we expanded the various stages of the cancer care pathway and sourced additional articles that would provide further patient quotes, e.g. around social care issues such as financial difficulties experienced by people affected by cancer. We consulted with Macmillan programme leads and heads of departments to identify as wide a range of references as possible. Next Jane Bradburn and Jane Maher suggested that we test the information with our patient and carer group to refine the quotes and check that the language was comfortable to them. (Lorraine Sloan, community facilitator)*

A further person involved at this stage was the organisational sponsor for both the Macmillan GP community and this patient group, Glyn Purland. He maintained close communication with the NHS Cancer Services Collaborative (CSC), so that the literature review took into account work already done on this subject by the CSC. We can see already that several conversations had taken place even before Lorraine started to work directly with the patients and carers in her group.

### Translating NHS lingo into everyday language

Next, Lorraine followed the two Janes' suggestion by exploring with the patient and carer group what kind of language ordinary people would relate to. The earliest drafts, based on the literature search, had contained a good deal of NHS lingo (doctorspeak and nursespeak). The group found its own ways of expressing many phrases – for example, instead of 'discharge from hospital' members came up with 'going home'; instead of 'rapid access to appropriate diagnostics', they chose 'people want their diagnosis to be made as quickly as possible'. As a result, one of the document's most distinctive features became the clear, everyday language used in it.

Group members also added their own further thoughts to the document, and took early versions to other groups they were involved with in various localities around Britain. In this way, they gathered a range of suggestions to improve the draft. For example, one member was part of a breast care focus group in Wales – a network of women who were concerned about the lack of emotional support for patients in the community. The issues they raised were passed back to Macmillan via Lorraine and helped to improve the draft further. (The person who told this story recalled later that, when *Our Principles of People-Centred Care* eventually came out, she had the pleasure of taking it back to the women who had been involved.)

Once the Macmillan patient and carer group was happy with the draft, Lorraine circulated it around Macmillan for further comments. After a final draft was agreed within the organisation, about 3000 copies were sent out with the magazine *MacVoice*, which was routinely distributed to Macmillan nurses, GPs and other professionals around the UK.

## SPREADING THEIR OWN WORDS

The example of *Our Principles of People-Centred Care* shows how the social life of documents can start with their creation, and this particular document had what might be termed a lively 'pre-publication social life'. But documents also continue to 'meet people' after they have been produced. To find out what kind of social life this one enjoyed after its first appearance, and whom it influenced, one of us attended a meeting of the patient and carer group that helped create it. We asked the 12 people there on the day to tell us how they had seen the document being used. We also explained that their stories and examples would be recorded and then used to compile a narrative account called 'The social life of a document', which they would be the first to see, comment on and help revise or expand. (See box for examples members gave us.)

### A document meets people living with cancer

*Our Principles of People-Centred Care* got an airing with people both inside and outside Macmillan. When we listened to the group, it was astonishing and encouraging to discover just how many arenas the thinking had found its way into – a true ripple effect. We transcribed these new stories in full and the excerpts below are in people's own words:

One member told us: 'I have my office in the Health Shop, which is a drop-in for wellbeing in north Norfolk, mainly for women but also for families. I put *Our Principles of People-Centred Care* up on my billboard and I used it to identify all the local services that Macmillan and others provided pertaining to each item. For example, next to "bereavement" I had a Priscilla Bacon leaflet, and I also had the Feeling Good thing that we provide locally, plus the Macmillan nurses, the Red Cross, and my support group. So I had a whole collage. It was a good journey for me to see what was actually relevant and what information I had. So if somebody phoned me up I would know'.

A second person said: 'I've given it to people with cancer whom I support. . . . They start talking about what they really want. . . . "That will actually help me put into words what I will say to my doctor". Quite a few families have had it – parents, older brothers and sisters, a couple of 13–14-year-olds have looked at it. . . . It puts into words quite simply what people are thinking about and perhaps what they've been through'.

We also heard how one member had seen *Our Principles of People-Centred Care* being used at a Macmillan meeting. People were talking about what the charity's priorities should be in planning its services and somebody went and fetched *Our Principles of People-Centred Care*. The member reported that a number of points were picked up from the document, which made the group feel very proud.

As well as proving useful to patients and carers, *Our Principles of People-Centred Care* found its way into the hands of many health professionals (*see* box).

**A document meets health professionals**

*Our Principles of People-Centred Care* was sent to all Macmillan professionals, including doctors, nurses, allied health professionals, other practitioners and researchers. In the first few months of 2004, numerous requests for further copies flowed in from all over England, including hospital cancer nurses, oncology and radiotherapy departments, and managers. The Department of Health received copies too.

We also came across anecdotal evidence that the document had a direct influence on hospitals. For example, one member reported that she had taken it to the core cancer team at her local hospital: 'These are professionals such as oncologists, people from the hospice, and lead nurses from the hospital, and there were volunteers like PALS [Patient Advice and Liaison Services] officers and so on in there too. . . . They were very interested in it and they want to translate it into standards for the hospital.' The same member gave it out to numerous local support groups, and also to a friend whose son was a consultant involved in educating nurses.

In another part of the country, the team reorganising a new cancer centre in Hertfordshire made use of *Our Principles of People-Centred Care*, potentially benefiting 4000 new cancer patients a year.

Finally, the patients and carers also told us many stories of the document being used directly in the training of health professionals.

***1 Nurse training***

One person said: 'I was invited along to talk to nurses going through their BA [Bachelor of Arts] and I used it as an aid. One of the girls asked if she could keep it, so I managed to get hold of others and I sent them all out. The last I heard it has been included in the portfolio for the girls going through their training. And it's also in the Cancer Centre in Aberdeen – up on the wall in the treatment room. They find it useful just to bring them back to normal reality, I think. It's an *aide-mémoire* about what the patient is going through and what he or she wants from them. The nurses found it easy to read, and it reminded them that a patient has feelings and this is what they want'.

***2 Other professional training***

Another commented: 'I used the poster version for two workshops. The first was on supportive communication in cancer care. That was with radiographers and other staff within X-ray departments, including nurses . . . they said they wanted to see the journey right through including the treatment and death/bereavement aspects. . . . The second workshop was on "embracing change" and was again for staff from X-ray departments. . . . I gave them [*Our Principles of People-Centred Care*] in its draft format and asked them "What do you think?" and they thought it was very good.'

We have seen that both the creation and dissemination of *Our Principles of People-Centred Care* depended on a range of human interactions and contributions. At the time of writing, the document lives on and continues to influence, and one key factor contributing to its success is the fact that it was created with extensive involvement of the very kinds of people who were likely to use it, in words they could relate to. These people also seemed eager to give it a social life.

There are striking similarities between this story and one featured in the book mentioned earlier, *The Social Life of Information*.[5] The authors relate how anthropologist Julian Orr studied Xerox technical representatives who were responsible for repairing copiers at customers' sites. At the time, the reps were provided with documentation about how to repair copiers, but this failed to help them when faced with non-routine problems or unpredictable machines. Following Orr's work, the company decided instead to create a new database called Eureka – the difference was that this time it was not a top-down creation, but one which grew out of the reps' own tips, refined through peer review. Reportedly, this tool became not only indispensable to them but it also provided recognition of the value of their creation and allowed knowledge to be shared between people located far apart.

Another factor helping to keep *Our Principles of People-Centred Care* in circulation was the fact that both Jane Maher and the community facilitator (Lorraine Sloan) remained in Macmillan throughout and were mindful of the need to keep the document alive by introducing it to key people.

## INTRODUCING DOCUMENTS TO HUMAN BEINGS

Pursuing the 'social life' metaphor a bit further, we have come to think of the 'introduction' as possibly the most significant act that enables a piece of writing to influence people and behaviour. An introduction can take any form – person to person, by phone, via email or web. If it happens during a conversation, clearly the introducer can take the opportunity to gauge the interest of the person listening and respond in the moment. If it is done via email, it is worth taking considerable care, e.g. by directing the email to just one person, enticing them to read (and share) the document by letting them know why they might find it interesting or useful, and indicating what kind of response they are being invited to give (perhaps you want them to comment on content or tone, but not to dot 'i's and cross 't's). It helps to know the communication preferences of the person receiving a document. Do they like to be contacted by phone or by email? If email, will an attachment be a stumbling block (e.g. if they are too busy to open it or if they are receiving the email on a mobile device, such as a Blackberry, i-phone or smartphone.)

**Perseverance sometimes required**

Making a successful introduction may need perseverance, as members of the patient and carer group mentioned earlier discovered:

'I took *Our Principles of People-Centred Care* to our cancer network meeting and there was a new facilitator – it was the second group she had run. I said at the end "Perhaps you could make copies and circulate them in the minutes". "Fine", she said . . . and that was the last I saw of it! I stupidly gave her all my copies apart from the one with everybody's amendments on it. I'm quite upset that nobody else has seen it, but I've just become the chair so I'm going to do something about it'. (person living with cancer)

'My GP surgery refuses to have any posters up. They've taken the copy I gave them and put it into this book of patient information. I asked them "What are you doing with all the information?" and they replied "We'll put it in this file that's kept under the desk". I've been going to that surgery for 31 years and I didn't even know about the file. I just keep talking to them and hope someone will see the light'. (person living with cancer)

We have experimented with putting documents on websites or wikis – some people are glad they can access items whenever they want to, and they do so; others simply do not visit the site. Perhaps this will change over time, but for now there is a wide variation in people's readiness to download documents, let alone read and respond to them.

The importance of giving documents an introduction brings us back to a central argument of this book, which is that, despite all the reports written and all of today's online communication, face-to-face conversation arguably remains the most effective way of influencing people. This is true even (or especially) in a world of overflowing email inboxes and mountains of 'pre-read' (papers circulated for study before meetings). There is something to be said for comparing informal introductions and conversations with 'just-in-time manufacturing'. This was a concept coined in the 1980s to describe a shift of emphasis from storing raw materials and parts to making them available 'just in time', thus speeding up production and saving costs. By analogy, conversations can be timed to influence someone just when it counts – in this sense, they can be highly efficient. Documents, on the other hand, are stored information which is time consuming to create. In this connection, we find Wenger's notion of 'accompanied artefacts' particularly compelling:

> *[I]t is often a good idea to have artefacts and people travel together. Accompanied artefacts stand a better chance of bridging practices. A document can give a less partial view of a topic, and a person can help interpret the document and negotiate its relevance. (Etienne Wenger)*[6]

Here we give an example of a piece of writing that became far more influential than it might otherwise have been, thanks to an introduction quite late in the day.

**How introductions helped an article become seminal**

The document in question was an article authored by a research fellow with a nursing background (Jo Armes), who went on to become a founding member of a Macmillan-sponsored community of influence focused on the effects of cancer and its treatment.

In healthcare and many other sectors, publication obviously matters. Specialist doctors and academics are expected to publish articles as a way of disseminating their evidence and helping to sustain the reputation and funding of their institution. The article we describe here came to be seen as seminal, but could easily have remained relatively obscure.

The article had many things going for it. To start with, it was the first systematic study in the UK of patient needs after cancer treatment. It was special in other ways too. The research was conducted by a number of nurse researchers, who were particularly excited about the project because, if nurses are involved in research, often it is in drug trials rather than in studies of the psychosocial aspects of patient care. Moreover, the researchers succeeded in involving a very large number of patients (the questionnaire was sent to 1850 people, with a response rate of 79% at the end of treatment and 62% after six months). No less than 66 centres were drawn in, compared to 20 expected. (These impressive figures were partly due to the fact that the study was 'NCRI-badged', meaning that any National Cancer Research Network nurse could recruit patients.)

The article was also a great example of collaboration – a blend of clinicians and researchers working together – and this contributed to its success. Each of the 10 named authors played an active role in the project: Professor Alison Richardson[7] and Maggie Crowe co-led it, others advised on the design of the research, while Jo Armes was the research fellow who managed and executed it, and a patient contributed a lay perspective.

The findings themselves were also significant: they revealed the extent to which the health service was failing to meet cancer patients' needs after treatment: 30% of patients reported more than five moderate or severe unmet needs. Furthermore, for 60% of these individuals, these needs (the most common of which were psychological problems and fear of recurrence) were still unmet six months after cancer treatment. The results suggested, in other words, that there was a proportion of survivors with unmet needs who might benefit from selective provision of psychosocial care.

The involvement of so many people in the research meant that the article enjoyed a lively social life during its creation. But it also encountered many people after publication. Its post-publication social life started out pretty much like any article appearing in a high-impact journal (in this case the US-based *Journal of Clinical Oncology*[8]). As lead author, Jo engaged in the usual activities to give the research wider academic and medical exposure, including speaking at professional conferences. And the timing of publication was favourable as the National Cancer Survivorship Initiative (NCSI) was just about to be launched in the UK. With a dearth of data about patient needs after treatment, the NCSI used the findings in its 'vision' document.[9]

Furthermore, the paper stood a good chance of influencing practice on the ground in the NHS. This was partly because, as we have seen, it was written by nurses – making it more likely that other nurses (the very professionals who are most likely to be able to meet the patient needs identified) would read and respond to it. Also, it clearly pointed to which kind of patients health professionals might support more actively in future (e.g. those with 'low-grade anxiety' – a condition that is rarely looked at in medical research, where people often focus on clinical depression).

Most significantly for the point of this story, the article had some determined 'introducers'. Alison Richardson made sure that English Cancer Czar Mike Richards received it. Jane Maher, as sponsor for the NCSI project group looking at consequences of cancer and its treatment, took special care to hand the article to anybody she met who was influential in the field. Nevertheless, it took some months after publication before it received widespread attention. It was after Jane Maher gave the article personally to Macmillan Chief Executive Ciaran Devane that he started to use it as a platform for his discussions about cancer survivorship. The chief executive's 'push' made all the difference – only then did people appear to start talking seriously about the research. Jo Armes later reflected:

'This was interesting to me because, as one of the authors, I was not party to discussions that were held about the paper within Macmillan. . . . To be honest, with the exception of [Jane Maher], no one at Macmillan had ever made any comments to me about the paper . . . I only became aware that Macmillan was using the paper because other researchers told me . . . I guess from my perspective, whilst the paper may have a "social life", it is not one that the authors have been asked to participate in.' (Jo Armes)

What we can see from this example is a document that enjoyed the kind of post-publication social life that is normal for articles in academic journals, in the sense that it was talked about at specialist conferences and circulated among the authors' contacts. But then, after some delay and without the authors' knowledge at the time, it was apparently given an 'introduction' that made it far more influential than it might otherwise have been. In effect, it went off on its own (without its parents) and met people. The story shows that authors are not always aware or kept informed about what happens to their own creations. Sometimes it is a third party who introduces the child to new friends. It is worth noting, finally, that introducers can increase the chances of documents being influential if they tell people something about how the document came into existence and what is special about it.

## REVIVING USEFUL DOCUMENTS

A good document created by a community sometimes has to rest a while before the time is right for it to be refreshed, revived or more widely adopted. The story of Macmillan's 'Out-of-hours toolkit'[10] is a case in point.As we saw in Chapter 3, the Macmillan GP community had highlighted out-of-hours care as a problem back in the early 2000s – when things go wrong for cancer patients, it is not always at 10 a.m. on a work day, and may be at 2 a.m. on a public holiday when their local practice is closed. A Macmillan GP wrote a report on the topic, published in 2001, and much of the thinking went into the Gold Standards Framework. However, out-of-hours care remained a nagging problem for the NHS and for many patients living with cancer. So about five years later, Macmillan decided to refresh the out-of-hours report by inviting the Macmillan GP community to engage with it during a 'speed-dating' exercise at one of their twice-yearly meetings.

**Using 'speed-dating' to refresh a report**

Speed-dating is a method normally employed in an entirely different context, where it involves single professional people meeting a large group of potential partners in one evening. They spend just a few minutes in conversation with each person and decide on the basis of that brief encounter who, if anyone, they might like to get to know better. We have used a similar process on a number of occasions, usually to bring together professionals and lay people to generate ideas on a particular issue, using it as a time-efficient form of brainstorming. In this particular case, we used 'speed-dating' to generate and collect problems and solutions related to out-of-hours care.[11]

Next, Macmillan GP Advisor Rosie Loftus and community facilitator Lorraine Sloan worked with Department of Health experts to put some of the learning into policy and practice. Among the outcomes at this stage were two new 'do not resuscitate' policies, which were subsequently adopted by the NHS. These were an important part of enabling patients who wanted to die at home to do so.

Despite the report and the perseverance of Rosie and Lorraine, the out-of-hours problem remained in the air and continued to be a theme for the GP community. To help address the continuing problem, therefore, Macmillan's GP Advisor group agreed to take it up yet again. What eventually emerged was the Macmillan 'Out-of-hours toolkit' mentioned above. Published in 2009, this offered guidance to all providers of out-of-hours care, and gave commissioners valuable evidence for their negotiations with providers. Macmillan disseminated thousands of copies through its website, CDs and paper versions. The toolkit also moved into the e-learning arena, being used in the education of multiple professionals responsible for out-of-hours care. And it was widely promoted and featured in a joint newsletter issued by Macmillan and the Department of Health's End-of-Life Care team.

What the story above shows is that, although much effort had gone into the earlier out-of-hours report, it was only later, when the Macmillan GP Advisors and others agreed that there was still work to be done, that the issue was readdressed. Although it took years to get there, publication of the Macmillan 'Out-of-hours toolkit' in 2009 was timely. Research published in that year suggested that 75% of patients still did not know whom to contact out-of-hours,[12] and there was also a national debate going on about giving dying cancer patients access to 24/7 care in the community.

## HOW LOOK AND FEEL CAN MAKE A DIFFERENCE

We want to draw attention finally to one more factor that can increase the chances of a document getting a social life. This is look and feel, which includes not just the language used, which we have already highlighted as important, but also layout and usability. The example of what happened to *Our Principles of People-Centred Care* shows how a certain amount of to-ing and fro-ing may be needed before people can settle on a look that is acceptable to all involved.

### A process of trial and error

*Our Principles of People-Centred Care* went through at least three different formats before settling down into one that people could agree on. The original request had been for Lorraine to condense the literature review into five or six bullet points defining people-centred care, but she rapidly came to the view that such an abstract summary would not be very useful. She started with a spreadsheet for collecting all the information, but eventually turned it into a folded A2 document (four times normal copier paper size) laying out the whole of the cancer journey in 10 stages, starting with prevention and early signs of cancer through treatment and beyond. In other words, the information was presented in the form of the 'patient journey' rather than boiling it down into an abstract list.

It is worth pausing to notice the judgement that Lorraine exercised here (a sound one in our view). There is a tendency in organisational life today to issue statements in condensed, bullet-point form. Sometimes this may be helpful but often the information just becomes vague and lifeless. What Lorraine did was to make the 'patient journey' the context and then present it as one large spread that could be taken in at a glance but also studied in detail.

Subsequently, Macmillan's corporate communications team worked with members of the patient and carer group to develop a design and layout for the next edition of *Our Principles of People-Centred Care*, with the intention of making it both practical for users and recognisable as a Macmillan document. The redesigned document that emerged ran to several A4-size pages and was intended as a middle way between poster size and something that would fit into a pocket or bag. At one of the group's meetings in 2004, this A4 version was handed round as a 'mock-up'. This prompted members to recount how they had been using the earlier poster-size version, suggesting that there was a need for more than one format. For example, some people might want an A4 version that would fit neatly into a training handout, but others might prefer a poster to hang on notice boards or use as a 'poster presentation'.

At time of writing, *Our Principles of People-Centred Care* had taken on yet another look – each page was A4 size but the whole document could be unfolded to show the entire cancer journey as one spread. This gave it the flexibility to be used either as a handout or as a poster.

Turning next to guidelines created by health professionals, the two stories below show how brevity is sometimes essential if good-practice advice is going to be used by professionals.

### A more usable version of a lengthy good-practice guide

*Cancer in Primary Care: a guide to good practice* started life in a workshop convened by Macmillan in 2002, led by National Cancer Director, Professor Mike Richards and involving a number of primary care professionals. As part of the consultation process, it was then tested with the PCCL community. The project was managed by Glyn Purland (organisational sponsor for the Macmillan Support Programme for PCCLs) and the final product ran to more than 50 pages, covering myriad aspects of cancer care, from health promotion and screening to supportive and bereavement care.[13]

Some Macmillan GPs spotted an opportunity to create a more concise and usable version. For example, GP Cathy Burton discussed what to do with the *Guide to good practice* with a multidisciplinary cancer group that she had helped to set up in London. They agreed that, if this were sent in its entirety to GPs, they wouldn't look at it. So they decided to distil it down and combine it with information about local and national resources. This took some time, with people working on separate sections between group meetings. The result, completed during 2004, was a four-pager known as *A Quick Reference Guide to Cancer in Primary Care*. Under four headings – Health Promotion; Screening; Early Diagnosis & Continuing Care; and Palliative Care – it laid out the main aspects to focus on and practical measures to take, and then provided relevant sources of information. The group produced a laminated version but also made it available electronically via the website of the local cancer network. Around 50 practices received this version, every practice manager getting between 10 and 20 copies, which they could pass on to GPs, practice nurses and other staff.

Similar short and user-friendly documents were created in other parts of the UK. For example, Macmillan GPs in Scotland put together some brief guidelines in the form of a desk blotter pad (at a time when many GPs still used a pen!), based on the official Scottish Referral Guidelines for Suspected Cancer. This was widely distributed and generally appreciated as a good reminder for busy practitioners of the symptoms and signs that required early referral for further investigation. Distilled versions were also incorporated in electronic information and referral systems used by general practitioners.

**Ten top tips – using a group's knowledge in a pragmatic way**

In 2009 Macmillan Cancer Support created a new community of influence (jointly funded by Macmillan and the Department of Health), known as the Consequences of Cancer Treatment collaborative group (CCaT). Like many groups, CCaT saw an opportunity to create some guidance for patients and/or professionals. Mindful that it can take months or even years to produce guidelines that are strictly evidence-based and widely tested, the group agreed it would be helpful to make a start by creating some user-friendly 'top tips' aimed at improving care for cancer survivors. In doing this, they were following the example of Macmillan GPs who had created similar documents (e.g. 'Ten top tips for palliative care', published in Macmillan's electronic newsletter for primary care professionals[14]).

As members of CCaT began teleconferencing and exchanging emails about what should go into their top tips, there was an understandable urge to produce a 'master template'. We reminded them that the point was to come up with a provisional set of top tips rather quickly by drawing on their collective experience, so that they had a 'good enough' first draft that could be tested and refined over time. They could continue compiling a 'master template', but meanwhile the provisional version would be of practical use and could have a productive social life, gathering feedback from a wide range of people.

These last two examples reveal something about the value of documents created by health professionals for health professionals. Perhaps only they fully appreciate the pressures on busy clinicians, who want key information at their finger tips – in concise format.

## POINTS TO CONSIDER WHEN GIVING WRITING A SOCIAL LIFE

Many useful guidelines have limited impact on practice, often because there are hurdles to overcome on the ground, e.g. inadequate dissemination, power/status issues or the infamous 'not invented here' syndrome. We offer some thoughts about how to increase the chances of useful written information influencing practice.

### Writing a document is just part of the work

As we have seen, communities of influence often choose to write down tips or guidelines based on collective knowledge and experience. This is to be encouraged, as long as they fully appreciate the need to give their products a social life both during their creation and after publication. One of the great advantages of text is that it can be revisited again and again to stimulate new conversations, learning and influence.

Furthermore, if guidelines are to influence behaviour, the ground may need warming up before they are spread, e.g. by testing what might prevent health professionals from adopting new practices.

### It matters who does the writing

It really makes a difference who contributes to the creation of documents intended to inform, educate and influence. A document's 'social life' begins when people work together to create something that they can feel they own and that will be useful to themselves and others in a similar situation. Ideally the people a document is written for (whether professionals or lay people) should have a hand in choosing the language and words used and identifying a user-friendly format. Top-down instructions tend to have limited use or influence.

### The part played by a community facilitator

Where a group or community of influence is creating a document (e.g. patient information, clinical guidelines), we have found it helps if there is a community facilitator who is able and willing to manage the process, working in collaboration with group members. In the case of the patient and carer group that helped to create *Our Principles of People-Centred Care*, the facilitator made sure diverse points of view went into the document. She also exercised her judgement in shaping and revising the document, while always remaining responsive to what the patient group wanted.

### Look and feel matter

How a document looks is much more than an aesthetic or cosmetic issue. Length, layout and language can all make the difference to whether busy health practitioners read and, most importantly, act upon it. There is a place for both long and short documents. Short guidelines and tips may stand a better chance of influencing behaviour. But sometimes longer reports are useful, e.g. for gathering evidence together or constructing what we referred to in Chapter 2 as a 'kitchen sink document' (one that can be drawn on or remodelled to create a more focused version for a specific set of readers when the need arises). A longer report may sometimes be necessary to document and demonstrate the importance of a particular issue.

### Reviving good documents when the time is right

People in organisations are always creating written information. Often, though, there are already really good documents – draft guidelines, unpublished articles, or unsuccessful funding proposals – that deserve to be revived. When the climate becomes more favourable, it is much more likely that the ideas expressed by the author will be taken up.

### Importance of a human being 'introducing' documents to key people

The fatal mistake that many make is to produce a document, publish it or send it to a number of people, and then sit back while others supposedly take it on board. The reality, as we probably all suspect, is that information and instructions are often ignored. The crucial move often comes when somebody who wants the document to make a difference – possibly but not necessarily the author(s) – gives it or sends it to key people, making clear why it is worth reading.

## NOTES

1 Brown JS, Duguid P. *The Social Life of Information.* Boston: Harvard Business School Press; 2000. The authors looked at the social context that gives information meaning.

2 Wenger E. *Communities of Practice: learning, meaning and identity.* Cambridge: Cambridge University Press; 1998. pp. 58–64.

3 Stacey R. *Complex Responsive Processes in Organizations: learning and knowledge creation.* London and New York: Routledge; 2001. p. 187.

4 Ong WJ. *Orality and Literacy.* London and New York: Routledge; 2002 (first published 1982 by Methuen & Co). p. 8.

5 Brown, Duguid, op. cit. pp. 99–113.

6 Wenger, op. cit. pp. 111–12.

7 Clinical Chair in Cancer Nursing and End of Life Care Southampton University Hospitals NHS Trust and the University of Southampton, Professor of Health Sciences at the University of Southampton.

8 Armes J, Crowe M, Colbourne L, *et al.* Patients' supportive care needs beyond the end of cancer treatment: a prospective, longitudinal survey. *Journal of Clinical Oncology.* 2009; **27**(36): 6172–9.

9 Available at: www.ncsi.org.uk/resources/ncsi-reports/ (accessed 19 April 2011).

10 Available at: http://be.macmillan.org.uk/be/s-209-toolkits.aspx (accessed 23 December 2010)

11 Lank E, Donaldson A, Maher J. Using the concept of speed dating in research into illness. *European Journal of Palliative Care.* 2008; **15**(1): 26–9.

12 See Sheldon H, Sizmur S. *An Evaluation of the National Cancer Survivorship Initiative Test Community Projects: report of the baseline patient experience survey.* Picker Institute Europe; 2009. Available at: www.ncsi.org.uk/wp-content/uploads/NSCI-Evaluation-Report.pdf (accessed 23 February 2011).

13 NHS Modernisation Agency, the NHS National Cancer Action Team and Macmillan Cancer Relief. *Cancer in Primary Care: a guide to good practice.* 2004.

14 'Macmillan primary care update'. June 2010. Available at: www.macmillan.org.uk/Aboutus/Healthprofessionals/Primary_care_cancer_leads/Resources.aspx (accessed 23 February 2011).

CHAPTER 5

# Hybrid creatures

## A novel way of bridging the gap between research and service improvement

### OVERVIEW

*In 2004, Macmillan formed a small group of 'hybrid creatures' – individuals with combined professional identities, all of whom had an interest and track record in working to improve services for people affected by cancer. The intention in forming this group was to test whether it could provide a model for academics with clinical backgrounds to do research that could be rapidly translated into service improvement, while also developing collaborative relationships over time. Although by now Macmillan had long experience of working with professional communities of influence, there was no template for a hybrid group of this kind. It therefore took considerable testing and negotiation before trust was established and results could be demonstrated. To provide an initial focus for this group, Macmillan invited members to conduct research into a framework designed to improve supportive care for cancer patients in the community.*

*At the time of writing, after some six years of working together, members of the hybrid researcher group had expanded their influence, created and disseminated useful evidence about supportive care, influenced education and training, developed helpful new tools, and generated further funding for research in this important field. This by now well-established group remains available to be called on by Macmillan and others to evaluate new services for people living with cancer.*

In the public sector, especially in healthcare, evidence is generally needed to evaluate the effectiveness of particular services or forms of care. The difficulty often is that researchers based solely in academic institutions may be too remote from practice, and constrained by the pressures of academic life, e.g. the need to publish constantly to boost their university's research ratings. Improving services on the ground is simply not their first priority. And even if they would like to see patient care improved, they may not have much influence over health professionals or policymakers.

From their perspective, organisations wanting to fund research that makes a difference may ask themselves both 'Is it useful?' and 'Is it cost-effective?'. They might have qualms on both counts: findings from academic research often take too long to appear to be timely for practitioners eager to test new services, and when the research is concluded, full-time academics typically take the knowledge they have accumulated back into their institutions. Moreover, research is expensive, especially where full-time university salaries need to be paid.

## TESTING A NEW APPROACH TO COLLABORATIVE RESEARCH

Starting in 2003, Macmillan started testing a novel approach to these issues by forming the Macmillan Palliative and Cancer Care Research Collaborative (MacPaCC).[1] The intention was to see what would happen if selected individuals were invited to work together over time in order to make research really useful to healthcare practice.

In focusing on 'hybrid creatures' (people with both clinical and academic identities), the expectation was that, although initially less senior or prominent than their full-time academic colleagues, such people would be dedicated to improving patient care. Moreover, their ongoing clinical responsibilities would keep them alive to patient needs, enable them to identify questions that needed researching, and take up ideas that emerged out of research and put them into practice. Finally, hybrid creatures, typically fluent in the languages of research, education, service development and clinical practice, would be well placed to build bridges and influence people in these somewhat separate domains. In other words, by working with hybrid creatures, Macmillan was 'designing in collaboration from the start'.

In general, academics and clinicians can be quite different types of people, with contrasting senses of urgency around healthcare improvement. Academics typically want to follow rigorous scientific procedures and get all the data collected and analysed before drawing conclusions or recommendations. Clinicians and service developers, on the other hand, characteristically want to test and spread new services as quickly as possible without waiting years for academic papers to be published.

In practice, MacPaCC members covered the whole spectrum – there was one full-time academic, one or two full-time clinicians, and some 'true hybrids' (health professionals with part-time academic posts). Over time, some members in a sense became more hybrid – for example, one nurse embarked on a PhD, while the full-time academic started new research projects evaluating services for patients.

### A joint inquiry: improving care in the last year of life

To give all these individuals (numbers fluctuated, but about 10 in total) an opportunity to collaborate over time, Macmillan invited them to start by focusing on a particular clinical issue within the field of end-of-life care.

The invitation to join the group was therefore rather specific: people were invited to work together to produce evidence to support the sustainable uptake and spread of the GSF (the Gold Standards Framework for supportive care for cancer patients in the community, introduced in Chapter 3) in the UK.[2]

When people think about cancer, their first association may be the treatments given by specialists in hospitals, e.g. surgery, radiotherapy and chemotherapy. In recent decades, however, there has been growing awareness of the need for supportive care provided 'in the community'. People sometimes refer to this as *primary palliative care*, as it is centred on the role of the GP, community nurses and other general practice staff looking after patients before and after hospital treatment. It includes, but is not limited to, end-of-life care. Historically, primary palliative care has been an under-researched field. An analysis published in 2002 by the UK's National Cancer Research Institute (NCRI) revealed that research into supportive and palliative care accounted for only about 4% of direct cancer research expenditure by NCRI partner funders (Department of Health, Cancer Research UK, Macmillan Cancer Support, Marie Curie Cancer Care, and the Medical Research Council).[3]

At the time the group was created in 2004, Macmillan had already invested a substantial sum (some £1 million) in encouraging the spread of GSF processes to hundreds of general practices across England and Northern Ireland. Furthermore, a flow of data was beginning to emerge out of the questionnaires filled in by practice staff, and Macmillan had commissioned the University of Warwick to lead a two-year programme evaluating GSF implementation. (One of the key researchers, Dan Munday, a palliative medicine consultant and former GP, became a founding member of the new group.)

The general consensus at this time was that the GSF was working, but more evidence was needed. Such evidence was not only important to improve implementation, it was also needed to justify including end-of-life care in the new GP contract being renegotiated at the time (the General Medical Services contract), which would in turn encourage general practices to pay more attention to this aspect of care. As we saw in Chapter 3, Quality Outcomes Framework (QOF) points (part of the performance management and incentive system for GPs in the UK) were later established for both keeping a register of people diagnosed with cancer and holding regular meetings to plan their care.

The point we are making here is that a 'joint inquiry' can give members of a group something to focus on – something that creates a sense of purpose in the early days, when people might otherwise be struggling to find a 'direction of travel' for their work together. Without such an inquiry (and even with it), they may be anxious to know the answer to questions like 'What are we supposed to be doing together? What does the funder expect? Where is this all going to lead?'. Some may feel nervous about investing time and achieving little more than 'just talk'.

What we have learned is that the funder needs not just to provide as much clarification as possible at the start, but also to offer plenty of opportunity during initial community meetings for members to develop their own sense of joint purpose – what do they care about, what do they want to influence collectively? However, in practice it doesn't seem to matter how hard the funder tries to articulate its priorities and objectives at the beginning – some members of a new group may still feel confused or frustrated in the early days. They may be used to the more familiar situation in which a research council or other funder issues a written brief and leaves researchers alone to develop and submit their proposals, which are then either accepted or rejected.

### How soon does a new group need a name?

A memorable name for a new community of influence can help to create a sense of an established group, something that people can 'point to'. In effect, a name can help to make the group more visible. In the first year or two of this group's life, people referred to it using the unwieldy title 'Macmillan GSF Research and Evaluation collaborative group'. After that, the group itself chose the name Macmillan Palliative and Cancer Care Research Collaborative (MacPaCC). Agreeing on a public name became important when members found they needed a logo to use on conference presentations and other publications.

## CULTIVATING AN INFLUENTIAL LEARNING COMMUNITY

The group that began to meet regularly from 2004 onwards represented five UK universities – Cambridge, Edinburgh, Huddersfield, Sheffield and Warwick. A sixth, Birmingham, joined the following year. In addition, the group included two people affected by cancer (one of whom was a patient and one a person who had lost her daughter to the disease). Other people also took part in community meetings, e.g. members of the funding organisation.

MacPaCC was presented explicitly with two overarching aims. As we have seen, it was expected to 'produce evidence to support the sustainable uptake and spread of the GSF in the UK', and also to 'act as a learning community to develop models for useful research and collaborative ways of working'. It is worth pausing to notice what was unusual about this second intention: the researchers were not just being asked to pursue relevant research, but also to help to test the concept of creating and sustaining a collaborative community of active researchers with clinical experience.

Some readers may wonder how the community of influence described here differs from the many other groupings in the NHS (e.g. networks and multidisciplinary teams). We think this question can be answered quite quickly: MacPaCC was not designed to *provide* one efficient, coordinated service. Instead it was created primarily to *influence*, by developing evidence for service improvements and pressing for advances in patient care.

Another term that is quite widespread in the NHS is 'interprofessional collaboration'. This has become important because, given increasing complexity in health and social services, there is a need for coordination and collaboration between professions and agencies. In a recent review of interprofessional collaboration, Leathard concluded that 'What everyone is really talking about is simply learning and working together'.[4] At this general level, there is a similarity with our communities of influence work. On closer inspection, however, there are some distinctions worth making. MacPaCC was *not primarily* 'interprofessional' in the sense of people from different professions or 'tribes' working together. Doubtless, in their workplaces MacPaCC members do need to influence various professionals, such as doctors, nurses and health visitors. However, what made this group distinctive, we think, is its *hybrid* nature – all core members bar one had clinical backgrounds as well as being research-active, making it easier for them to work across professional barriers.

### Building on a web of existing relationships

Often when organisations form working groups, taskforces or committees, they issue an invitation to tender for membership and then endeavour to judge applicants on merit. This is designed to guard against the risk of the group being just a collection of somebody's cronies. With communities of influence, the situation is a special one. A capacity to collaborate and influence depends crucially on being able to develop and nurture relationships. It is not surprising then that pre-existing relationships – among group members as well as with the funding organisation – are to be viewed as an asset. In any case, given that people are typically chosen for their interest in a specific issue, they tend to know one another already, or at least *know of* each other.

Thus, when approaching people who might be interested in becoming founding members of the new collaborative research group, the Macmillan team naturally wanted people with a relevant track record in the field. But it was equally interested in individuals who had long-term relationships with it, as sponsoring organisation, or with each other. (These criteria were stated explicitly in documentation drawn up in the first year by the senior manager who held the budget for the group.)

**Who knew whom?**

Many members of MacPaCC had a considerable history (with the inevitable mix of experiences) of working with Macmillan and the Macmillan GP community. This meant there was less need to spend a large amount of time explaining Macmillan's ways of working. Some founding members had particularly long-term links with the charity. For example, Bill Noble (consultant in palliative medicine and former GP) had been connected with it since 1996, when he was appointed Macmillan Senior Lecturer in Palliative Medicine at the University of Sheffield. Stephen Barclay from Cambridge (see written portrait below) had been one of the earliest Macmillan GPs, beginning a three-year appointment as a 'Macmillan GP Facilitator' in 1995. (*See* Chapters 1 and 3 for more about these Macmillan professionals, referred to more generally in this book as 'Macmillan GPs'.)

Most members had also been closely connected in the past with the GSF. Virtually everyone knew Keri Thomas, who had developed and piloted it. Many had already worked with her, either as fellow researchers, or (in one case) as her academic supervisor. And the first nurse to join the group (Jane Melvin), was the Lead Nurse for the Macmillan GSF spread programme in the UK.

## PORTRAIT OF AN INFLUENTIAL CLINICIAN RESEARCHER

The story of one member of the group – GP academic Dr Stephen Barclay – helps to bring alive the notion of a 'hybrid creature' and some of the tensions the multiple identity can entail.

Stephen's interest in palliative care went back to early life experiences. His mother had died when he was just seven, and later, as a medical student in Oxford, he worked in a hospice. Then in the 1980s, as a GP in a rural community, he saw the benefits of using a 'hospital-at-home' service to support patients dying at home. It was when he moved to Cambridge in 1989 that his interest in research was awakened. There he joined a practice that had a long tradition of teaching and research and he made contacts with academics specialised in palliative care.

Stephen continued to pursue his interest in palliative care by taking up a three-year part-time post as 'Macmillan GP Facilitator' in 1995. This gave him a few hours of protected time each week to develop his palliative care skills and test ways of providing education and advice to other GPs. In his last 12 months in this post, he embarked on a survey of GPs and District Nurses in the Cambridge area, which alerted him to the different perspectives of these two groups around palliative care and laid the ground for later, wider-scale research.

In 2002, he resumed collaboration with Macmillan by taking up a new three-year post as Macmillan Clinical Fellow. This gave him a day and a half per week to provide academic support to Macmillan GPs, teach medical students in palliative care, and develop his own programme of research in this field. His academic base was at the General Practice and Primary Care Research Unit, part of the University of Cambridge and led by Professor Ann Louise Kinmonth. Throughout his fellowship, Stephen benefited from periodic meetings in Cambridge, where representatives of Macmillan (including Jane Maher) and the University explored how they could best support him and make his fellowship a success. There were tensions involved in pursuing a combined clinical and academic career, but these meetings seem to have helped:

### 'At the interface between oil and water'

> *The first few discussions weren't easy. We didn't know each other and I felt that I was at the interface between oil and water, between a five-star academic unit and a service development charity. However, I've had strong support from both Ann Louise Kinmonth and Jane Maher. (Stephen Barclay)*

The first meeting also put him in touch with one of Macmillan's most influential GPs, Rosie Loftus, who became a strong ally and helped him extend his research by embarking on a major study involving more than 1000 GPs and 500 District Nurses across London and southeast England. Thirteen Macmillan GPs were involved as researchers; this was a rare opportunity for GPs to participate in such work, and the fact that questionnaires came from peers facilitated good response rates (around 60%). The research led by Stephen generated recommendations about roles in palliative care, which could influence policymaking.

When MacPaCC came into existence, Stephen was a natural candidate, and his participation in the group became one of the agreed objectives/elements of his Macmillan Clinical Fellowship. Asked later how MacPaCC had been useful to him, he emphasised the value of being 'part of a supportive peer group' where he could regularly bounce and debate ideas in a 'friendly but not uncritical' environment. One memorable occasion occurred in 2006, when the group helped him rehearse his interview for a highly competitive Department of Health postdoctoral research fellowship (funded by Macmillan). Not long afterwards he was awarded the fellowship, giving him five years to pursue a programme of research focused on understanding patient preferences in primary palliative care.

At time of writing, Stephen was some four years into the fellowship and was on sabbatical from his general practice in Cambridge. Nevertheless, he maintained his 'hybrid' status, keeping in touch with patient needs by continuing to work regularly on-call for the local hospice. In June 2010 he learned that he had succeeded in his application for a permanent academic post at the University of Cambridge. This allowed him to continue combining research, teaching and clinical GP work.

### Value of being a hybrid creature in a hybrid group

A number of themes emerge from Stephen's story – for example, how a hybrid creature can act as a bridge, moving freely between the worlds of research, education and clinical practice; how a long-term three-way relationship between a doctor, a university and a charity can bear fruit; and how membership in a collaborative R&D group can be a source of support to the individual as well as providing an opportunity to become more connected and influential in a field that matters to patients. In his own words, Stephen Barclay summarised his relationship with Macmillan as a sponsoring organisation as follows.

> *I would never have got to this point without the long-term support I have had from Macmillan, going back now over 15 years since I started as Macmillan GP Facilitator way back in 1995. . . . Over the years that Macmillan has supported MacPaCC, all have had academic positions strengthened. . . . Macmillan is unique in the way [it] supports clinicians to develop as academics while maintaining their clinical roots. (Stephen Barclay)*

Stephen's contributions included not just invaluable evidence on how primary care practices can best look after cancer patients but also the influential position he developed, especially in education (*see* boxes).

#### Sharing knowledge and evidence

*Publications:* Stephen Barclay published dozens of articles or editorials as first author and several as joint author with other members of MacPaCC, in journals including: *British Journal of General Practice*, *European Journal of Cancer Care*, *Journal of Pain and Symptom Management*, *Palliative Medicine*, and *Journal of Cancer Nursing*. Many of these publications enabled him to continue 'harvesting' his MD thesis and thus influence thinking in the field of primary palliative care.

*Presentations:* Made to a range of organisations and conferences, including the Royal College of General Practitioners, Society for Academic Primary Care, United Kingdom Conference of Educational Advisors, Macmillan GP conferences, and University of Glasgow Palliative Care Congress.

*Data and knowledge shared:* With other members of MacPaCC, including data from the survey of 1000 GPs and 700 District Nurses, and the literature survey from his MD thesis on General Practitioner Provision of Palliative Care.

*Academic base established in the field of palliative care:* Stephen played a leading part in creating a new palliative care research group in his academic unit in Cambridge, helping to establish recognition for the unit in this field, attracting substantial research funding (more than £800 000 at the time of writing), and employing six researchers.

**Influence on education and policy**

Stephen also made contributions to practice and education. For example, he enabled many GPs to develop a better understanding of research and evidence. With today's emphasis on evidence-based medicine, it is important for doctors to be able to assess evidence and understand how to apply research findings to their clinical work.

He also helped to give palliative care a more prominent place in medical education. By working together with colleagues at his academic unit, Stephen helped expand the palliative care component of the new curriculum of the University of Cambridge School for Clinical Medicine. He was subsequently appointed Specialty Director for Palliative Medicine at the University and at the time of writing continues to teach there. Medical students in their final year see two dying patients, which means that they really engage with supportive care – not in a hospice setting, but in the 'messy reality of the community'.

In addition, Stephen provided valuable evidence for policy. For example, in his doctoral research, he found that GPs were generally over-optimistic when predicting life expectancy of cancer patients in the last year of life. This meant that some patients were missing out on benefits as people were fast-tracked into the benefits system only if their GP declared that they had less than six months to live. Stephen's findings gave Macmillan's policy team extra evidence to campaign for the government to change the lead-in time from six months to one year, which has yet to happen, but with around 139 000 cancer deaths annually in England and Wales, the potential beneficiaries are numerous.

### Embodying the concept of the hybrid creature

Looking back, it becomes clear how valuable it was to identify an individual who embodied the concept of 'hybrid creature'. Stephen was a real person who could be pointed to, to exemplify what such a creature can do. The protected time that Macmillan funding gave him helped him to achieve some major tangible results.

The fact that we provide a portrait of Stephen Barclay should not detract from the many achievements of other hybrid creatures in the group. For example, Bill Noble was able to use his protected time to develop a new palliative care service in his part of England – the funding provided by the Macmillan regional team provided a locum to take over his clinical responsibilities for some hours each week. This new service made it possible to attract a senior registrar to take up a previously unattractive post as palliative medicine consultant. Similarly, Dan Munday was able to use his protected time both to finish his PhD and to develop a team of healthcare assistants specialised in end-of-life care in his own region.

## TRACKING PROGRESS OF A GROUP FROM THE START

Compared with the GP community, where we started the narrative tracking some years into its existence, with MacPaCC we had the advantage of being there from the beginning. Thus, over the first three years (2004–07) we convened and participated in MacPaCC meetings and drafted six separate accounts describing aspects of the group's evolution. These were: the story of its early life; two individual portraits (one clinician researcher and one lay person); an account of the negotiations around money; and two papers intended to attract continuing support from the funding organisation. The narrative accounts 'captured' otherwise ephemeral conversations and stories, thus 'making the invisible visible'. They also helped the group win continued funding after the first three years were up.

As in all our narrative evaluation work, we deliberately included considerable detail in the narrative writing, consistent with our premise that change and influence emerge from the 'messy detail' of human interaction (*see* Chapter 2). For example, in MacPaCC's case, we gave specific examples of some of the activities going on between community meetings: members had exchanged comments via email about study proposals, participated in one another's project steering groups, and had met up at key national events and visited one another at their respective universities to discuss particular studies. We found that such conversations between meetings were worth encouraging and tracking.

More than six years after MacPaCC's creation, the narrative record also enabled us to go back to the very first months and remind ourselves of issues and concerns that were arising then and may have been half forgotten since. These may well be relevant to other groups. Among the issues alive in the early parts of the MacPaCC story, five stand out as particularly relevant for any organisation seeking to establish a new community of influence (*see* box).

### Issues that may trouble group members in early days

***Will we be able to get on with 'real work'?***

On the whole, hybrid creatures juggle many different responsibilities, so they are eager to use their time together productively. Indeed, we have found that clinician researchers are at their most enthusiastic and energetic when talking about nitty-gritty research issues, such as the challenges in wording survey questions or the time taken to obtain ethics approval. They probably find such topics more compelling than managerial activities such as objective setting or funding arrangements. We remained convinced, nevertheless, of the value of allowing time in the early days for members to get to know one another, work out what connects them and agree a 'direction of travel'. To satisfy the desire to get on with 'real work', we started to allocate a growing proportion of time in community meetings to 'open space'. This meant that on the first evening of a one and a half-day meeting, people had an opportunity to make bids for time to talk about issues emerging around their research on day two.

***How about academic freedom and impartiality?***

Academics are naturally concerned about their freedom to look at evidence without being constrained by the needs and priorities of the funding organisation. In the case of MacPaCC, some members expressed a concern early on that Macmillan might be expecting them to 'prove the effectiveness of one particular intervention'. The Macmillan people present were able to ease these anxieties by stating clearly that the researchers were not being asked to 'prove' anything, but simply to describe and explain – they were free to report weaknesses of the GSF as well as its strengths. 'Negative results are terribly important;' said one Macmillan person, 'if a development programme doesn't work, or if elements of it are not working, we need to know.'

***Is the funder committed for the long term?***

Anyone joining a collaborative group may ask themselves 'How committed is the funding organisation? Is it worth investing time and effort here?' In the first year, MacPaCC members raised questions of this kind and the budget-holding manager was able to reassure them that he would be applying for an extension after the initial two-year commitment. This, along with the offer of project funding, seemed sufficient to convince them that this was a serious investment by Macmillan in developing a collaborative research community.

***Who is in and who is out?***

Even if not spoken out loud, one potential issue in groups is nearly always membership ('Who is in, who is out, who has the most influence?'). Collaborative research groups are no exception. People continue participating in a community of influence as long as it feels mutually useful, and this makes such groups different from teams within a management structure. No individual can be expected to commit indefinitely to participate, and at any one time some may feel more committed and enthusiastic than others. With MacPaCC we tried to keep this question open: members agreed that some fluidity was a good thing and that when new members were introduced they needed appropriate 'induction' to understand the group's way of working. After six years, most of the original clinician researcher members remained in the group, and it had succeeded in integrating a number of new ones as well as strengthening the nursing presence in the group.

***Can I speak my mind freely?***

Finally, confidentiality is a concern that commonly arises in any new group, especially if its conversations are being recorded and 'tracked' by a narrative writer. Members may wonder whether they can feel free to speak their mind in community meetings, whether they will have a chance to influence the written account, and how it will be used. In the case of MacPaCC, agreement emerged quite early on that the first narrative account would remain an 'inside story' and successive drafts would therefore be distributed only to members of the group. If members wished to circulate drafts to further people (here we gave examples of who these might be), this would be agreed by the group, and the person receiving the draft would be asked to treat it as confidential. Should anyone want to create an external publication related to MacPaCC's work, this would be discussed and agreed collectively.

We concluded it was well worth making time for open discussions about issues like group membership, confidentiality and academic freedom. Researchers and funding organisations naturally face different pressures and priorities and it is best to give these an airing from time to time.

As time went on, further fundamental questions arose that will be relevant to many groups – for example, will people (in this case, academics) from different institutions collaborate, what value is there in involving lay people, and what does it cost to keep people round the table? Below we explore each of these important questions in turn.

## WILL ACADEMICS SHARE AND COLLABORATE?

There are barriers to knowledge sharing in every organisation. Common ones include the 'not invented here' syndrome, competition for resources, organisational 'silos', company culture, business processes and technology.[5,6] Where academic institutions are involved, there may be additional hurdles to overcome. Indeed, we have heard it said that academics 'never really collaborate'. They may feel a need to keep their unpublished research to themselves; they may be anxious about ownership and getting credit for it; and they are typically under pressure to contribute to boosting their own university's research ratings. Yet, as soon as a group of clinician researchers comes into existence, there will be useful resources that can be shared – skills, knowledge, project proposals, data, service improvement ideas, publications and so on. The pooling of these resources may even be one of the group's first tangible achievements. We found again that open discussion at community meetings helped to ease anxiety. The following story illustrates how, despite all these tensions, sharing can happen.

### Taking a gamble on sharing knowledge

In MacPaCC's first year, Stephen was on the verge of submitting his MD thesis, so his literature review was a natural candidate for sharing with other members of the group. The review itself was about 70 pages long and represented a substantial amount of work and accumulated knowledge. At a meeting in his academic unit in Cambridge, two main concerns were raised about the suggestion of sharing his literature review with other MacPaCC members: (i) that publishers could object, and (ii) that someone could use some of the insights without attributing them. Nevertheless, it was agreed that he would put his views about this to the next group meeting. A note circulated before the meeting emphasised the benefits of collaboration, while hinting at potential barriers:

'I think we have real potential for undertaking some very significant research work together that can fill some of the big gaps in our knowledge concerning palliative care in primary care, which in turn can improve care for patients, which is what we are all about at the end of the day. But we also need to acknowledge the need to develop our own research careers, and we are all mindful of the agendas of our institutions'. (Stephen Barclay)

At the group meeting, members initially discussed the option of Macmillan funding a completely new literature review, but concluded that this would not be a good use of money. Instead, after some discussion, Stephen agreed to act as a test case by circulating his own review, to stay strictly within the group. In doing this, he felt he was 'taking a gamble'. At the end of the discussion, he commented:

'Talking openly about this was great. We are past talking about collaboration now, we are now doing collaboration'. (Stephen Barclay)

The example above highlights the time it can take to achieve the trust and openness needed for a group to act as an effective community of influence.

## WHAT CONTRIBUTION CAN LAY PEOPLE MAKE?

Two lay members took part in MacPaCC. After a few months, one (a cancer patient) was unable to continue on health grounds – inevitably this can and does occur from time to time. However, the other lay member stayed on and became a long-term member of the group. A common concern about 'user involvement' is that it will either be 'tokenistic', or that lay members will be given too much voice or push their personal hobby horses. Roberta Lovick's story below shows that this need not be so.

### Roberta becomes an advocate for research

In the years before Roberta Lovick joined MacPaCC, she had lost her daughter to cancer and cared for a number of sick people close to her. Her history as a volunteer with Macmillan pre-dated the MacPaCC story, so she had some relevant experience before joining the group.

Her first encounter with researchers, in 2003, had not been easy: when she attended a meeting in London that year as part of a group of lay people helping Macmillan Cancer Support develop its work with doctors, she was surprised by what she experienced:

'I was upset because the researchers were on one level having coffee and we were sent to another room to have coffee, and I felt that that was quite strange . . . because how can we change things together if we're separated at the initial meeting?' (Roberta Lovick)

A few months later Roberta took part in a follow-up meeting in Bristol, focused on user involvement in research. This time lay people outnumbered professionals and she had another striking experience as she listened to the researchers:

'I sat with one of the patients, and she wrote something on a piece of paper and shoved it across to me. It was just a scribbled note saying "I thought research was to do with drugs. Am I wrong?" Well, that was what was going through my mind, so I thought *Here goes*, and I actually put the point . . . and from us saying that we thought it was drugs-related, the researchers realised that they needed to help and teach us a lot more, which they did.'

It was shortly after the Bristol meeting that MacPaCC was formed. Roberta was invited to take part in the meetings from the beginning. Typically she would sit quietly for long periods and then ask a disarmingly direct question. With time, she became increasingly articulate and bold in her participation, which was informed by her many conversations with patients, carers and clinicians. When we spoke to her, she was able to look back and say that the barriers she had experienced earlier no longer existed for her. Also, she had become so conscious of why research matters, that outside the group she often found herself arguing the case for GPs being actively involved in it.

As well as participating in MacPaCC meetings, Roberta was invited to be part of the 'commissioning group', sitting alongside senior managers and sharing the responsibility for reviewing research proposals and making sure they were linked to patient benefit. This was a mark of everyone's confidence in her ability to contribute her experience as a carer when evaluating research ideas. On more than one occasion, Roberta was asked directly for her view on specific proposals. For example, did she think the subject of end-of-life care in nursing homes was important to service users? And did the research proposal being put forward by group members on the subject make sense to her? Her answer to both questions was yes. She felt that people in care homes were often 'getting a raw deal, and that this needed to be researched'.

One of the difficulties for any lay person participating in a group of researchers is that the language and concepts can seem foreign, at least to begin with. At one group meeting where people were talking about their research proposals, Roberta, who had read the relevant proposal (on the role of community nursing), asked them to clarify something. As a result, the two people proposing this project went on to create a lay summary, which Roberta welcomed:

'The proposal was extremely difficult for me to understand and, although I did persevere with it and read it several times . . . the minute I got the lay summary I sent my answer back to say it was fine and that I'd had an answer to my question.'

Reflecting on her experience of working with the clinician researchers, Roberta described how she got used to speaking up:

'I find every meeting difficult . . . I have to pay lots of attention and I suppose I always worry that somebody's going to put me on the spot and ask me something that I don't understand . . . and the more I thought about it, the more I thought, well, patients may be in the same situation where they need to be able to say "Could you explain that?" Often, patients come out of a consultation and really do not understand what has just been said to them . . .'

'. . . I go to all these things hoping that somehow or other all of us can make a difference for the next generation. And sometimes you've got less than five minutes within a whole meeting, which might take a day, to do that. So you have to pluck up the courage to actually do something about it. If you really feel moved by something, you have to make that effort to say something.'

Gradually, Roberta came to think that a key part of her contribution was to 'bring the researchers back to earth':

'I could sit and swallow a dictionary and know all the terms and understand them as much as the people around the table, but then I wouldn't be looking at it from the normal patient's or carer's point of view.'

Roberta's story demonstrates the value of maintaining a long-term relationship between lay person, funder and group, as well as some of the pitfalls to look out for when inviting members of the public to join discussions with academics or healthcare professionals. After experiencing Roberta's presence in discussions, Macmillan's then head of research remarked that he had no sense that she pursued her own personal agenda. Indeed, he became more convinced than ever that service-user involvement grounded what Macmillan did, stressing that 'if something doesn't make sense to service users then it's not worth doing'.

## WHAT DOES IT COST TO KEEP PEOPLE ROUND THE TABLE?

Every funder wants to get value for money. One common approach is therefore to issue an open invitation to organisations or individuals wanting to tender for research funding. In such cases, the relationship with researchers typically remains arm's-length and document-driven. With a community of influence, there are good reasons for making the relationship between group members and funder a closer one. First, a group of this kind is not just about funding specific projects, but is an investment in relationships over time. Second, we found that an ongoing dialogue between the two parties helped to shape research projects that would contribute to improving services. In some ways charitable funders like Macmillan are less like research councils and more like commercial organisations, in that they need knowledge in order to develop and improve products and services. It makes little sense for them to allocate funding solely or even primarily on the basis of scientific excellence and academic prestige.

**Different types of funding**

In the case of MacPaCC, different types of funding were needed to 'keep people round the table'.

*Group-based funding:* Including travel, accommodation, and administrative support (*c.*20% of the total).

*Person-based funding*: This element (protected time or 'backfill') was designed to free up members of the group from their normal responsibilities, for a given number of days per year, so they would have time to work with one another and with Macmillan Cancer Support. The amount and form of payment was tailored to individual circumstances (*c.*30%).

*Project-based funding:* Macmillan also offered funding to pursue research, publication and collaboration (*c.*50%).

With the project funding in particular, the Macmillan team wanted to test a collaborative approach to commissioning, to find out whether this would provide 'reach and impact' – in other words, significant benefits for people living with cancer. To begin with, the team drew inspiration from the notion of 'iterative commissioning' developed by Richard Lilford and colleagues.[7] However, it very much tested its own approach, making modifications as it went along, so the commissioning process evolved over time (*see* box).

**Project funding: a collaborative approach**

Though every project was slightly different, the commissioning process that emerged can be described in general stages, as follows.

1 *An initial brief:* Macmillan developed a broad brief indicating the topics it wanted to

have researched. The overall topic was implementation and impact of the GSF, with a few specific questions identified.

2 *Research ideas generated by researchers:* Usually in the form of draft outline research proposals.
3 *Commissioning group:* Macmillan formed a special commissioning group to allocate the project funding, help the researchers refine their proposals and link them clearly to patient benefit. It included a senior manager as decision-maker, with other members taking an advisory role. As we have seen, lay member Roberta Lovick played an influential part in setting priorities, assessing bids and clarifying patient outcomes. All members of the commissioning group also participated in MacPaCC's regular community meetings.
4 *Dialogue:* The work of the commissioning group consisted of starting a dialogue with the researchers to tease out specific research questions and agree on research methods. Some negotiations took place via email, some face-to-face, and some by teleconference. Often these discussions prompted researchers to modify their original proposals.
5 *Commissioning brief:* Macmillan developed the practice of responding to proposals by writing its own brief to record the results of the above discussions, filling in any gaps it saw in terms of research outcomes, service-user involvement, etc. The aim was to reframe the researchers' proposals and take other people's views into account (e.g. other members of MacPaCC). In other words, the commissioning brief was an attempt to reconcile the proposed research project with the purpose of the group and the strategic aims of the funding organisation.
6 *Range of outcomes specified:* Instead of relying just on a standard research report, Macmillan specified exactly what outcomes it wanted from the research. They varied widely, e.g. a syllabus for a training course; an article in a specific publication; a specification for a service; or suggestions for refining an intervention.
7 *Continuing dialogue:* The commissioning brief gave the researchers approval in principle (the 'pale green light'). The 'to and fro' then continued until there was reconciliation between Macmillan's brief and what the researchers felt was doable.
8 *Formal grant letter:* Once the grant was formally approved, the university in question could move things forward, e.g. by advertising for research assistants, where appropriate.
9 *Staged funding:* Because the kind of research being described was hard to specify in detail and in advance, funding was staged with continuing review. If necessary, proposals could be modified again as research progressed.

How did the clinician researchers react to this collaborative funding process? One commented that she was initially puzzled over its 'back-to-front' nature. She was used to funders providing detailed briefing documents and then leaving academics to draft their proposals. As we have just seen, there was only a broad brief to begin with. The formal 'commissioning brief' was drawn up *after* initial talks between the commissioning group and the researchers.

## MULTIPERSPECTIVE STORY: TALKING MONEY

The account within the box looks at one particular set of funding negotiations, preserving various perspectives in order to give a realistic sense of how the three main parties felt.

### Three takes on the same set of events

In April 2005, two of the MacPaCC clinician researchers jointly submitted an outline proposal to carry out studies into care planning at different stages of the cancer patient's illness. They were Stephen Barclay at the University of Cambridge and Scott Murray at the University of Edinburgh. The fact that the application came jointly from two universities instead of one was new for this group, but the researchers felt it was in keeping with the spirit of collaboration being encouraged by the funder.

Discussions had been going on for about two months when there was a difficult teleconference about the sum to be awarded. Macmillan's initial offer was for £80 000 over two years, which was less than the £100 000 requested. By all accounts, however, this call was a turning point. Once Glyn Purland, who held the budget for this group, had further clarification of what exactly the two researchers had in mind (i.e. employ two research assistants to free up time for the principal researchers to undertake specific pieces of work together), he agreed to try to find the extra funds.

After the call, the commissioning group finalised the brief, specifying precise outcomes expected. While the original proposal had defined only four general research outputs, the commissioning group expanded these to nine, including one on publications. The two researchers eventually got the sum they had asked for. Altogether the negotiations had taken some four months.

#### *Macmillan senior manager's perspective*

Glyn Purland had many years' experience working in the NHS. He felt that the process of iteration has significantly improved the research proposal and understanding between the researchers and the commissioners. However, for him, the full meaning of 'iterative' emerged only from several rounds of conversation:

> *We are all learning. It has only become possible to articulate what iterative commissioning*

*looks like in reality after learning from the negotiations around the first two or three projects. A process can only be defined and written down in practical detail retrospectively. (Glyn Purland)*

### *Clinician researchers' perspective*

The main sticking points for the two researchers were: (i) disappointment at the initial sum of money offered, and (ii) the time taken up with the negotiations:

*We had wanted for some years to do some research together and felt that collaboration between Edinburgh and Cambridge would be enormously fruitful, and members of the group encouraged us to take this opportunity to cement a relationship that had been growing over a number of years. We therefore thought we would do something slightly different from the other members of the group by applying jointly for £100 000 for a two-year collaboration. In April 2005, we submitted a four-page research proposal along these lines and the commissioning group then asked us to produce a one-page version for the group to discuss at its June 2005 meeting. We were slightly dismayed at that meeting to get a sense that we would not be awarded the full amount we were asking for. What happened was that another university (Birmingham) had come on board and made an application for a research project, in response to a need identified by the group. We felt it was terrific to have Birmingham coming on board, but this inevitably meant an extra demand on the original £250 000 budget. (Stephen Barclay and Scott Murray)*

The two clinician researchers reflected that the delay and uncertainty had been 'a bit frustrating'. Nevertheless, they stressed that the support from Macmillan was very welcome and that it provided funding that might otherwise not have been available for the kind of work they wanted to undertake (collaboration between two researchers, dissemination of earlier research, as well as a pilot study):

*It is difficult to get funding for this sort of thing. . . . Although my unit in Cambridge is very supportive, I work solo as a primary palliative care researcher there, so having a research colleague will make a huge difference and will also be an important signal to the unit. (Stephen Barclay)*

*The main attraction for me was the opportunity to disseminate some of the research findings from Scotland and the feeling that Macmillan might be interested in acting upon them. (Scott Murray)*

### *Chief Medical Officer's perspective*

Finally, Jane Maher's comments as Macmillan's Chief Medical Officer underline once more a key feature of the funding approach: that this was an investment in long-term relationships in order to influence practice in the health sector. It was also a new approach for all concerned:

*I see this as an investment in two individuals and their collaboration, rather than just in a project. . . . The traditional position of an academic applying for a grant is to get as much money as possible out of funders and tell them as little as possible. And there is often a lack of transparency around the commissioning process – for example, people have to hide things (e.g. producing publications) within the overall grant. . . . The negotiations are not easy for me. I know, though, that discomfort is normal when you are in a new situation, and what we are trying to do is new and different. (Jane Maher)*

The multiperspective story above clearly shows three different takes on the same set of events. The issue of funding always has the potential to generate strong feelings, and the people involved here were strikingly open about a process that had its raw moments.

**Further insights about research funding**

The multiperspective story about money also surfaces a number of more specific themes and principles in relation to the funding of communities of influence.

*Value (and rarity) of funding for certain research-related activities:* Such as collaborative behaviour, pilot studies and dissemination.

*Challenge of articulating outcomes from collaborative working:* The time needed for the commissioning group to feel satisfied that it fully understood what the money was to be used for.

*Importance of specifying relevance of research to patient experience:* The emphasis on identifying and documenting the kind of evidence needed to improve patient care before the funding was agreed.

*Investment in long-term relationships:* The aim was to invest not just in research but also in ongoing relationships with influential clinician researchers, so extra time was needed for dialogue and negotiation.

## WHAT'S IN IT FOR THE MAIN STAKEHOLDERS?

In the MacPaCC story, there were three main types of stakeholders (the clinician researchers, their employers, and Macmillan as funding organisation), all of whom needed to see some value in the group, otherwise it would have been unsustainable. Below we look at each of these perspectives in turn.

### Clinician researchers' perspective

At time of writing, all founding members of MacPaCC (bar one) remain actively involved in the group, suggesting that they see value in continuing membership. When asked, they reported benefiting from being part of a supportive researcher community as well as receiving funding to enable them to collaborate and undertake relevant research. Moreover, they developed a collective voice to press for improvements in practice and policy, not only by publishing and presenting their findings, but also by participating in influential bodies in the world of palliative care. For example, Bill Noble was appointed chair of the Association of Palliative Medicine (APM), and Scott Murray joined the APM's executive committee to promote the primary care agenda. Scott Murray and Stephen Barclay became co-chairs of the NCRI's subgroup on primary palliative care. Furthermore, three of the clinician researchers linked to Macmillan (Stephen Barclay, Dan Munday, Bill Noble) were all 'Named Collaborators' in one of the two NCRI collaboratives mentioned earlier. And finally, Keri Thomas left the group after the first year to dedicate more of her time to her role as clinical lead for the NHS End-of-Life Care Programme.

Our narrative tracking of MacPaCC ended in 2007, just as it entered a second phase of work and new managers took responsibility for its funding. However, while drafting this chapter in 2010, one of us had a chance to join a MacPaCC meeting to get a sense of how the group has developed since. It was striking how smoothly and swiftly members at this meeting got down to sharing nitty-gritty detail about their research. For example, one pair shared methodological issues by setting up a role play (a patient–doctor interaction). All in all, this was clearly a well-established group enjoying productive time together.

### Host universities' perspective

As the second stakeholder, the universities had to be satisfied that their employees' involvement in the group was of value to an academic institution. The most obvious measure of that was the individual's contribution to the university's research rating. The numerous peer-reviewed publications produced, often as a collaboration between two or more members of the group, were a clear enough outcome. More generally, some university department heads needed to feel reasonably certain that their people 'were not collaborating their lives away' (as one put it). With about four community meetings a year (involving travel to and from the University of Warwick), and additional time spent collaborating and influencing in between meetings, the commitment was a significant one.

One researcher expressed the tension he felt in being part of a triangular arrangement. His university was driven by the research ratings that all UK universities have to submit to, whereas Macmillan was focused on improving cancer services. So inevitably he felt he was measured against two completely different criteria – almost inevitable for a hybrid creature.

Most members of the group felt well able to keep their university satisfied. For example, when he joined MacPaCC, Nigel King's situation as Reader in Psychology at the University of Huddersfield gave him considerable discretion in how to use his time. Although Macmillan had no formal connection with Huddersfield, he clearly felt able to participate in the group. While a member of MacPaCC he was appointed professor at the university.

One factor that proved particularly helpful to Stephen was the regular meetings set up to support his Macmillan Clinical Fellowship, attended by both Macmillan and Professor Kinmonth, his unit head, who indicated that the meetings helped her to see the value of Stephen's involvement in MacPaCC:

> *It is important for Stephen to be linked with others at the cutting edge in his field. Collaborative groups like this one give him that connection. . . . What's special is the link between research and service development. There are many groups who claim such a link, but I believe this one. You've built something very precious. (Ann Louise Kinmonth)*

### Funding organisation's perspective

Macmillan's fundamental expectation was that this community could help it pursue its strategic objectives – namely, to develop services and improve the experience of people living with cancer.

First, the projects undertaken by the researchers produced a wealth of evidence and knowledge about supportive care. The work also shed important new light on change in the NHS, demonstrating, for example, that processes may be implemented and evaluated quickly, but that changes in behaviour and relationships take much longer and are equally important to track. One by one, the six studies added to knowledge about: (i) whether process change can be equated to 'real' change; (ii) whether this kind of change is sustainable; and (iii) what makes an organisation such as a general practice receptive to improved processes.

Second, it was not necessary to wait years before reaping the benefits of this joint inquiry, as is often the case with academic research. Although it did take some five years before the definitive article on impact of the GSF was published,[8] in the meantime group members were able to draw on the findings as they emerged. Moreover, key decision-makers (e.g. National Cancer Director Mike Richards) were aware that these findings would soon be published.

Third, the funding organisation could turn to the clinician researchers, with whom it had an ongoing relationship, to help it evaluate new supportive care services – whether these were developed by the NHS, by Macmillan itself, or by a combination of the two. This sort of research is difficult to fund from other sources, especially in the development phases, yet it can bring real benefit to people living with cancer (*see* example in box).

**Community members at the ready to evaluate a new service**

The story of one particular study illustrates well the value of the lasting working relationships formed in a community of influence. In 2009, two particular MacPaCC members, who had not known one another before the group was born, made a successful joint bid to evaluate a new service in a rural area near Midhurst in southern England to provide supportive care outside hospital. After a few years of participating in MacPaCC, the two clinician researchers felt that they knew one another well enough for smooth collaboration ('we are on the same wavelength').

The two researchers' recent experiences were complementary and relevant to this project: Dr Bill Noble (Sheffield-based) had completed the national survey of palliative care in the community mentioned earlier, while Professor Nigel King (Huddersfield-based) had studied the relationships and tensions among the people involved in supportive care in the community.

The study was able to make use of a tool developed by Dr Noble for scoring general practices in terms of how likely they are to take up new processes. This was important because one of the questions that needed addressing was: 'Are the excellent results being achieved in the Midhurst area (e.g. 60% of deaths occurring at home, which is where most patients want to die) attributable to the new service itself or to the characteristics of the general practices working with it?'

Finally, the 'Midhurst study' was an unusual example of cooperation between a charity (Macmillan), two clinician researchers and a firm of management consultants. The Monitor Company's experience of collecting business data made it possible to obtain certain types of information (e.g. on cost of the service) relatively quickly. Thus there was no need to wait for the other parts of the study, which would inevitably be slowed down by lengthy ethics procedures or by the time needed to investigate complex phenomena such as working relationships and organisational context.

Added together, the total investment in MacPaCC over the first three years, including all the research commissioned from six universities in that period, was more than half a million pounds. Although this was a substantial sum, it was less than other collaborative ventures in the health sector. For example, not long ago, the NCRI – a partnership between government, industry and charity, with Macmillan Cancer Support being one of the 'member organisations' – set up a scheme for two Supportive and Palliative Care Research Collaboratives, with initial funding of £5 million over five years, starting in 2006.[9] In other words, NCRI partners were investing on average £1 million a year in two groups. Though hard to compare, since they are different kinds of collaboration, the point is that MacPaCC was relatively cost-effective. Above all, the research was well integrated with practice, and the funder could see and audit the links between research and service development. Finally, personal contact with the researchers was ongoing, whereas other funders are more likely to be reliant on the research report if they want to study detailed findings.

## TAKING STOCK: EVIDENCE FOR PRACTICE

In public and private sector alike, people are often anxious to know what the 'outcomes' of any endeavour are going to be *before* it is possible to specify them. With communities of influence, many of the outcomes emerge over a number of years. When we took stock of MacPaCC's achievements after three years of its existence, in 2007, it was clear that it had produced not only valuable evidence but also useful tools and methodologies for future research, and this in turn had helped members attract further funding for research in the field of supportive care. The MacPaCC projects funded by Macmillan between 2004 and 2007 are listed below, with lead researchers – all members of the group – in brackets. In the comments column, we show how one thing led to another – each study raised new questions that could be taken up in further research. All the projects were part of MacPaCC's 'joint inquiry' into the implementation and spread of the GSF.

**TABLE 5.1** Evidence produced in MacPaCC's first three years

| Project | Comments |
|---|---|
| 1 GSF national audit study (Dan Munday, Warwick Medical School) | This before-and-after study generated evidence of large-scale change in GSF processes taken up by general practices, e.g. out of 955 practices surveyed, the proportion having a 'palliative care register' rose from 23% to 90% between 2003 and 2005. This indicated that it was possible to spread processes around the NHS that were associated with positive patient experience.[10] |
| 2 In-depth study of GSF implementation (Dan Munday) | The audit served its purpose but more knowledge was needed, especially about the meaningfulness of the 'process measures'. There were two particular concerns: were the responses to the questionnaires 'real', and was the process change linked clearly to behaviour change? To explore these questions, the same team undertook a qualitative study looking at 15 practices in depth, comparing questionnaire responses with direct observation. This demonstrated that: (i) questionnaire responses and observation tallied; and (ii) process change had been sustained in most practices that had implemented the GSF. In addition, it indicated that effective palliative care requires not just robust processes but also good team relationships, especially between GPs and district nurses.[11] (NHS restructuring has since put GPs and district nurses into separate organisations, which may effectively inhibit the kind of casual encounters that help build relationships.) |

| Project | Comments |
|---|---|
| 2 In-depth study of GSF implementation (*cont.*) | And finally, the researchers investigated the value of having 'GSF Facilitators' (typically doctors or nurses) when introducing new processes, rather than simply providing practices with documentation and training materials.[12] |
| 3 National survey of general practices in the UK (Bill Noble, University of Sheffield) | The next study helped to reveal the bigger picture of 'what else was going on in primary care at the time?' The GSF was not the only set of tools designed to help general practices support patients near the end of their life – others included the Liverpool Care Pathway. So, one question that needed answering was 'Would the changes have happened anyway, without the GSF?' The national survey therefore looked at uptake of various processes. It was carried out one year after introduction of 'QOF points' for palliative care (these are points that influence remuneration paid to general practices), and found higher than expected uptake of the GSF (61% of practices overall, 80% in Scotland).[13] |
| 4 GSF in care homes (Collette Clifford, University of Birmingham) | The three studies described so far had focused on general practice. There was consensus in the group that it was also important to study the care given in residential homes. In this study, therefore, the researchers undertook a questionnaire survey of 49 homes. This indicated several improvements after GSF was implemented, including falls in both crisis hospital admissions and deaths in hospital. Communication between care home and GP proved particularly important for successful implementation. On the whole, use of the GSF seemed to have improved working relationships.[14] |
| 5 Understanding community nursing roles in primary palliative care – what are nurses doing on the ground? (Nigel King and Jane Melvin, University of Huddersfield) | The next study took up the relationship theme highlighted by the in-depth study (2, above), particularly the importance of the generalist nurse (e.g. community matron) in caring for patients near the end of life. The researchers pursued this further by means of 40 in-depth interviews with primary care teams in three parts of England, looking at the roles of community matron, district nurse and palliative care nurse. The research confirmed the central role of the generalist community nurse in palliative care, but also revealed some confusion around various nursing roles.[15] |
| 6 Ongoing collaborative research into end-of-life care – filling gaps in the evidence base (Stephen Barclay and Scott Murray, Universities of Cambridge and Edinburgh) | This 'project' was different from the others, in that the funding was intended to facilitate collaboration between two universities, including activities that are difficult to fund from other sources. Two research assistants were employed, one in Cambridge and one in Edinburgh, enabling the researchers to create new project proposals. This helped to develop a strong research programme in Edinburgh, which included recruiting two ESRC PhD-ships and securing substantial further grants for research into supportive care. |

These valuable MacPaCC products emerged from the group over a considerable period, demonstrating once more that funding organisations must be willing to make initial investments in a community of influence before exact outcomes can be articulated. This requires a leap of faith and a long-term commitment to the group that many organisations find difficult in a target-focused, measurement-driven environment.

### Tools and methodologies

The research projects undertaken raised further issues, and the researchers developed useful tools to address these. For example, Dan Munday's research drew attention to the influence of organisational context and relationships on the effectiveness of process change. In response, Nigel King and Jane Melvin developed a visual tool ('Pictor'), which enables people (e.g. health professionals, patients or carers) to map the relationships that play a part in their experience of care.

Dan's research also highlighted that practices need to be not only well organised but also 'receptive to improvement'. In response, Bill Noble developed the tool mentioned earlier, which helped researchers score general practices as good, medium and poor in terms of receptiveness to the GSF.

### Funding for further research

In the same period, members also played a significant part in securing additional grants from other major funding bodies for research into supportive care. Notable examples include a grant of more than £400 000 obtained from the National Institute of Health Research by three members of the group (Drs Barclay, Munday and Murray) for a three-year study with other colleagues on 'Definition and evaluation of models of primary and secondary care collaboration in end-of-life care provision'. Many other smaller but substantial grants were obtained by group members.

### Preparing the ground for a national initiative

Since MacPaCC members had already developed collaborative ways of working, they were in a good position to contribute to the new National Cancer Survivorship Initiative (NCSI) launched by the UK government in 2008 – for example, by undertaking evaluations of services being developed for cancer survivors.

The NCSI also prompted the Macmillan team to use the lessons learned with MacPaCC to help it create a further group of 'hybrid creatures', this time focused on the negative consequences of cancer treatment.[16] This was the Consequences of Cancer Treatment collaborative group that created the 'Ten top tips for cancer survivors', mentioned in Chapter 4. It consisted of 12 clinician researchers, predominantly senior nurses, all committed to improving care in this particular field.

## POINTS TO CONSIDER WHEN FORMING A HYBRID COMMUNITY

With the MacPaCC example, we have tried to tell a story that reveals both the substantial achievements of the group and some of the hurdles along the way. Below we offer some final thoughts to others who want to form their own hybrid group in order to use research to improve services.

### Identifying hybrid creatures

Perhaps the first question is, which kinds of 'hybrid creature' would benefit from being part of a community and become more influential as a result? The health sector has many people with combined identities – for example, managers and service developers with clinical backgrounds. Other sectors have their own hybrid creatures, such as researchers with a background in teaching, social work or other professions. In fact, any group of individuals who speak the languages of more than one discipline may have the potential to bridge gaps, develop a collective voice and influence practice and policy.

### What issue to focus on

Which 'joint inquiry' could such a group take on? Considerable exploration and negotiation may be necessary and useful in the early stages of the new group's life to clarify the focus of its work. It is counter-productive – and futile – to impose a task or focus on a group as though it were a normal project team.

### Funding arrangements

What funding arrangements will help support collaboration? The person holding the budget for the group needs to be somebody who really understands the spirit of a community of influence and the need to maintain a dialogue with group members (not acting as traditional funder at a distance). It may make sense for them to take part in community meetings.

### Maintaining the backing of employers

Hybrid creatures tend to have complex employment arrangements with several employers or stakeholders involved. It makes sense to think about what could be done to cultivate links with these participating organisations. It is important, for example, to ensure that the hybrid creature's employer (whether a university or a healthcare organisation) sees the value of the collaborative group and is reassured that the individual is not pulled in too many different directions.

### Lay involvement

Will there be lay members in the group? If so, it may take time and some support before they 'find their voice'. We found that involving a lay member in commissioning discussions helped ensure that the projects funded were shaped to address real patient needs.

## NOTES

1 Members of MacPaCC, 2004–07

| **Clinician researchers** | **University** |
|---|---|
| Dr Stephen Barclay | Cambridge |
| Professor Collette Clifford | Birmingham |
| Professor Nigel King | Huddersfield |
| Jane Melvin | Huddersfield |
| Dr Dan Munday | Warwick |
| Dr Scott Murray | Edinburgh |
| Dr Bill Noble | Sheffield |
| | |
| *Lay members* | |
| Roberta Lovick | Carer |
| Ray Strachan | Patient |
| | |
| *From Macmillan Cancer Support* | |
| Jim Elliott | Head of research |
| Jane Maher | Chief Medical Officer |
| Glyn Purland | Senior manager (budget holder) |
| Janice Koistinen | Macmillan Projects Support Manager |
| | |
| *Support ('learning framework' team)* | |
| Alison Donaldson | Writer |
| Elizabeth Lank | Expert in collaborative working |

N.B. This list includes those who were full members of the group and attended most meetings between 2004 and 2007. Since 2007, MacPaCC has absorbed a number of additional members.

2 www.goldstandardsframework.nhs.uk/ (23 December 2010).

3 www.compasscollaborative.com/ (23 December 2010).

4 Leathard A. *Interprofessional Collaboration: from policy to practice in health and social care.* Hove and New York: Brunner-Routledge; 2003. p. 5.

5 Lank E. *Collaborative Advantage: how organizations win by working together.* Basingstoke: Palgrave Macmillan; 2006.

6 Collison C, Parcell G. *Learning to Fly: practical knowledge management from leading and learning organizations.* Chichester: Capston/Wiley; 2004.

7 Lilford R, Jecock R, Shaw H, *et al.* Commissioning health services research: an iterative method. *Journal of Health Services Research & Policy.* 1999; **4**(3): 164–7.

8 Dale J, Petrova M, Munday D, Koistinen-Harris J, Lall R, Thomas K. A national facilitation project to improve primary palliative care: impact of the Gold Standards Framework on process and self-ratings of quality. *Quality and Safety in Health Care.* 2009; **18**: 174–80.

9 www.ncri.org.uk (23 December 2010).

10 Ibid. For a review of several GSF studies see also: Shaw KL, Clifford C, Thomas K, *et al.* Improving end-of-life care: a critical review of the Gold Standards Framework in primary care. *Palliative Medicine.* 2010; **24**(3): 317–29.

11 Munday, Mahmood, op. cit.

12 Petrova M, Dale J, Munday D, *et al.* The role and impact of facilitators in primary care: findings from the implementation of the Gold Standards Framework for palliative care. *Family Practice.* 2010; **27**: 38–47.

13 Hughes PM, Bath PA, Ahmed N, Noble B. What progress has been made towards implementing national guidance on end of life care? A national survey of UK general practices. *Palliative Medicine.* 2010; **24**(1): 68–78.

14 Badger F, Clifford C, Hewison A, Thomas K. An evaluation of the implementation of a programme to improve end-of-life care in nursing homes. *Palliative Medicine.* 2009; **23**(6): 502–11.

15 King N, Melvin J, Ashby J, *et al.* Community palliative care: role perception. *British Journal of Community Nursing.* 2010; **15**(2): 91–8.

16 See Donaldson A. A community of influence: clinician researchers join to make a difference to people affected by consequences of cancer treatment. In: Suchman A, Sluyter D, Williamson P. *Leading Change in Healthcare: transforming organizations using complexity, positive psychology and relationship-centred care.* Oxford and New York: Radcliffe Publishing; 2011.

**CHAPTER 6**

# Cultivating a lively community

## The role of the supporting team in helping a group become more influential

### OVERVIEW

*There are many practical ways of supporting and sustaining groups and communities, not least of which is having a well-balanced 'supporting team' in place, including some or all of the following: (i) a community facilitator; (ii) a community administrator/coordinator; (iii) an organisational sponsor; and (iv) a clinical lead. One further ingredient that proved helpful in our experience was what we call a 'distilling-and-connecting group' (mentioned in Chapter 3). Most larger communities of influence will have a core of very active members who invest time and effort in shaping community activities, and sometimes it is helpful to formalise the role of these members into such a 'community within a community'.*

*The ingredients above can make all the difference to maintaining a lively and influential community. Together the supporting team and the distilling-and-connecting group help to select and involve community members, clarify the purpose of the community, make community meetings productive, keep people connected between meetings, and last but not least, secure and maintain the funding needed to keep meetings and projects going. Without them, the community may lose its sense of direction, its momentum and its capacity to influence.*

A community of influence cannot be 'managed' like a normal team or working group, but nor is it realistic to expect such a group to be entirely self-sustaining. Even where members are committed and have a shared purpose, we have found that communities do need coordination and encouragement. Macmillan has always set up a supporting team for this purpose, involving several different roles. We start by looking at the community facilitator.

## COMMUNITY FACILITATOR: A VITAL CONNECTOR

*facilitate: to make easier the progress of (Collins free online dictionary)*[1]

This dictionary definition of 'facilitate' is very simple and general. In organisational life, however, the term 'facilitator' is more specific, often referring to someone who is responsible for designing and running satisfying meetings. Certainly the facilitators whose stories we tell in this chapter do tend to take responsibility for making community meetings productive and constructive. However, it takes a special kind of person to keep a community energised and engaged with its influencing work, so the community facilitators described here are much more than meeting facilitators (*see* box).

### Community facilitator: a wide-ranging role

*Connector over time:* Community facilitators do whatever they can to encourage communication and progress between meetings, to keep 'their' community focused and energised over time.

*Partner:* They build a strong relationship with the organisational sponsor(s), so that the community's credibility and contribution continues to be visible and valued across the funding organisation.

*Midwife or catalyst for creating knowledge products:* Where community members work together to create tangible products – such as booklets and guidelines – the facilitator can help to bring these into the world, enabling communities to capture some of their experience and share it more widely.

*Project manager (as needed):* While community facilitators are 'people people' first and foremost, in some situations it can also be helpful for them to have programme or project management skills, especially when tangible initiatives emerge out of the community they are responsible for.

*Translator:* Last but not least, facilitators act as bridge-builders or translators between group members on the one hand and other interested parties on the other. To pursue the translation metaphor a bit further, they do not generally do a 'literal translation'. Instead they make themselves familiar with the languages of the different stakeholders, e.g. community members and the sponsoring managers – and when necessary interpret between the two.

An example of a facilitator performing the 'translator' role (*see* box) is Lorraine Sloan (first introduced in Chapter 2). Lorraine was particularly skilled at talking to members of Macmillan's regional teams in a language they understood. The backing of these teams was crucial for the Macmillan GP community to retain its 'permission to exist'. On one occasion, Lorraine found a particularly creative way of helping them understand the nature and value of the community: first, she had conversations with several management stakeholders, and then she used some of their words in a paper about the GP community, which she presented back to the managers. Effectively she 'reframed' what she knew about the community in a way that managers could relate to. This kind of reframing can be crucial because, in many organisations, managers are sceptical or suspicious of communities and groups that are not on the organisation chart.

It will be obvious by now that community facilitation is not an administrative job. Indeed, administrative problems can seriously detract from the role. As we shall see later in this chapter, there is a strong case for bringing in a separate person with administrative skills to leave the facilitator free to focus on people, relationships and influencing.

## STORIES FROM COMMUNITY FACILITATORS

Here we provide three examples of people who facilitated different types of communities, all funded by the Department of Health and/or by Macmillan Cancer Support.

### Example 1: Lorraine Sloan – reconciling the priorities of lay people and doctors

Community facilitator Lorraine Sloan supported the Macmillan GP community for many years (and continued to do so at the time of writing) and became skilled in all the aspects of the role. From 2003, she also took on the facilitator role for a group of 15 patients and carers, set up to ensure that Macmillan's work with doctors was grounded in the priorities of people living with cancer.

Macmillan's approach to community building is especially interesting in that, whereas community members are *not* employees of the organisation, community facilitators like Lorraine *are* Macmillan employees (or people the charity pays to do this work). This is different from the NHS and many private sector communities, where both facilitators and members are generally employees.

In the case of the lay group of patients and carers, Lorraine was a crucial link between group members on the one hand and Macmillan and the Macmillan GP community on the other. Next we look more closely at how she developed her role.

### Supporting group members

Lorraine supported the patient and carer group in a number of ways. First, she organised and facilitated the community meetings, which were generally held every six to eight weeks. A typical gathering started at 11 a.m. with coffee. But before the meeting, people had the opportunity to gather informally and chat freely. Then, the meeting itself usually began with a reflection on what had happened since the last one. The next part of the day was typically more focused on future activities of the group that might facilitate Macmillan's work with doctors or improve the way Macmillan was working with people living with cancer. Then from mid afternoon, there was further opportunity for informal discussion.

During these sessions, Lorraine captured priorities raised by the group so she could identify which ones were also priorities for Macmillan and doctors. Her role was as much about connecting the group's ideas to relevant parts of Macmillan (and beyond) as about focusing on the patients and carers themselves. So she took care to help people understand Macmillan's agenda and to explain why the organisation was pursuing certain pieces of work over others. In doing so, she learned that people living with cancer did not see the organisation as divided into departments – in their eyes, the community facilitator represented 'all of Macmillan'. Also, they were interested in everything that Macmillan could do to improve things for people living with cancer, not just the aspects currently at the top of the charity's agenda.

One of the difficulties Lorraine faced with the group in its early life was a pragmatic one. Delays experienced in booking travel and claiming expenses were causing tension within the group. Expense claims often got stuck in the system and the process of reimbursement was variable across the organisation. She found that handling the nitty-gritty discussions on expenses as well as organising travel for people was taking up a huge amount of her time and detracting from her role as facilitator. During one particular meeting, the whole agenda became focused on the difficulties that individuals were experiencing in administrative support from Macmillan. Macmillan's Head of User Involvement, Jane Bradburn, who was familiar with such difficulties, advised Lorraine to ensure that she had adequate administrative backup in future. Once a dedicated administrative person had been identified for the group (*see* 'Lizzie Smith' story later in this chapter), Lorraine was able to focus on what she needed to do.

### Enabling the group to articulate the meaning of 'people-centred care'

Another valuable aspect of the role emerged when Lorraine helped the same patient and carer group produce the document *Our Principles of People-Centred Care* (introduced in Chapter 4). It took someone with Lorraine's energy and perseverance to make sure that a 'knowledge product' like this document saw the light of day. The result was a valuable and long-lived piece of literature created by service users for service users, in a language they understood.

### Encouraging partnership with GP community

As well as all the above activities, Lorraine also supported the group's members when they joined the twice-yearly Macmillan GP meetings, where their role was to work in partnership with Macmillan and its medical community. Often, the night before such meetings, there was an opportunity for the patients and carers to get together so they could clarify issues they wanted to articulate at the larger meeting and 'find their voice' before mingling with the doctors. Once they joined the GPs' conversations, one challenge for Lorraine was to make sure that the people living with cancer were not perceived as having an axe to grind:

> *I have learned the importance of the patient and carer group keeping the focus on partnership working – on things that are important for Macmillan, patients and carers, and doctors. But where possible I still try to give people a way forward for things which they feel passionate about, even if something cannot be taken forward as one of the group's priorities. (Lorraine Sloan)*

In other words, Lorraine was concerned to make sure that all participants in the meeting felt that their views were valued, even if they were not a high priority for others.

Asked what skills a community facilitator needed, Lorraine particularly stressed flexibility and adaptability – the art of dealing with emotional issues as they arise, knowing when to challenge and when to support. Facilitation cannot be approached as a mere task, she added; it requires empathy and the skills to build and maintain good personal relationships. Equally, in order to help service users navigate their way through Macmillan, Lorraine needed to know who was doing what across the organisation. And finally, she discovered the need to be patient, as involving service users can sometimes slow down progress. But, she added, 'it is invaluable if the work is to be truly grounded in the priorities of people living with cancer'.

After a number of years as community facilitator, Lorraine's role grew to encompass a considerable amount of programme management – this tends to happen naturally as initiatives originating in community conversations turn into major programmes of work. This means that, as well as being good at connecting people, facilitators will almost certainly need to have or develop programme management skills and be confident in high-level meetings. For example, Lorraine often found herself in meetings with senior managers within Macmillan, seeking the support needed to spread GP-led service improvement initiatives. And in 2010 she took part in meetings with the UK government to discuss how Macmillan's GP community could support a national initiative to improve early detection and awareness of cancer.

### Example 2: Beverley Roberts – a facilitator of facilitators across the NHS

In 2002 the Department of Health and Macmillan Cancer Support set up a joint initiative, the Cancer Partnership Project, the aim of which was to develop 'partnership groups' linked to the 34 cancer networks in England. These groups brought together patients and carers to work with healthcare professionals to improve cancer care. In effect, they provided a pool of service users who could contribute by helping to develop patient information, attend 'site-specific tumour groups' (e.g. breast, bowel) and shape the strategic priorities of the networks. Macmillan took an active part by setting up a Support and Advocacy Programme to develop and sustain the partnership groups.

Earlier experience in this field had shown that, for user groups to work effectively with health professionals, they needed facilitators, so the Cancer Partnership Project funded a facilitator for each cancer network in England. These individuals were paid employees from a variety of backgrounds who could, for example, help to bridge the gaps between lay and professional experience, as well as ensuring continuity when members were indisposed, e.g. because they were in full-time work or unwell. The facilitators were in turn supported by a Macmillan employee, Beverley Roberts, who effectively became a facilitator for a community of facilitators.

#### Developing skills that the facilitators wanted

Beverley's responsibilities included organising regional training days for the facilitators based on needs they themselves identified. The first round of these events gave them an opportunity to talk about how their roles were going. Discussions and subsequent evaluation showed that the facilitators had built up a good understanding of how to develop user involvement but they also faced a number of challenges, such as dealing with difficult group behaviour. They were therefore given help with understanding group dynamics. A second round of regional events provided an opportunity for facilitators to network and also to meet Macmillan staff who could support them.

### Bringing together partnership groups from around the country

Beverley also ran an annual meeting for all the facilitators nationally, which in turn informed the continuing development of user involvement and training in the NHS. The facilitators had further opportunities to meet nationally at the NHS-funded Network Development Programme days, which were good occasions to influence at a high level – for example, by putting questions to National Cancer Director Mike Richards.

### Winning over their managers

Beverley developed a relationship with the facilitators' managers, usually the lead nurses of the local cancer networks. This improved coordination and helped create a supportive environment for the facilitators.

### Establishing the role of facilitator

From Macmillan's point of view, investing in a lead facilitator not only made rapid sharing of good ideas easier but also helped to develop the facilitator role across the UK. Beverley's job continued for two years – it was never planned as a permanent one. Ultimately, the facilitator role became well established in the cancer networks and the facilitators went on to organise their own events. In other words, this proved to be both a useful and sustainable way of working.

## Example 3: Lisa Godfrey – flexible facilitator for NHS service improvement leads

In 2001, what was then the NHS Modernisation Agency had the task of streamlining the patient's journey through cancer diagnosis and treatment, using a methodology that had been piloted a couple of years earlier. The aim was to spread the methodology and learning to the 34 NHS cancer networks across England.

As part of this initiative, 34 'service improvement leads' were appointed, one for each network. The role of supporting the SIL community fell to Lisa Godfrey, one of nine 'service improvement regional directors' within the Modernisation Agency, who took it up with enthusiasm. As she put it herself, she 'fundamentally believed in the value of connecting people'. Below is an account of what happened.

### Initial enthusiasm followed by loss of continuity

The first priority was to develop the skills of this diverse group of people. The SILs were invited to come together twice a month for whole-day meetings – once for a meeting focused on delivery and once for a session dedicated to personal and role development. Lisa organised and facilitated these meetings and there was generally a good turnout. She cared about the group and felt she was there to support them.

When Lisa went on maternity leave, different people picked up the community facilitator role but over time attendance at SIL events fell off. The number of meetings was reduced and there was some criticism that the group had failed to meet expectations. Lisa reflected on the reasons:

> *This might in part be due to not having continuity in the facilitator role, but also I think principles and objectives need to be shared and owned at the outset, together with a shared understanding of what the group can and can't do. (Lisa Godfrey)*

### 'London story' unfolding in parallel

Meanwhile, reorganisation within the service improvement structure had reduced the number of regions from nine to four, one of which was the London area. The five SILs in London had established themselves as a subcommunity and were meeting every four to six weeks. Lisa initially chaired this group, although over time it became largely self-managed, choosing for example to rotate the chair role each time it met. However, Lisa continued to provide the group with advice and guidance as requested (often via phone) – for example, on how to become influential. She also helped to welcome new members to the group. And finally, she managed an annual budget of £50 000 to fund initiatives, which the London SILs could apply for.

Lisa commented that the London group created a safe space for people to work through issues and also acted as a support and 'action learning' group. It was sustained through several staff changes – thanks, in her view, to its modest size, local nature and shared issues.

### National group shifts from learning towards 'delivery'

Meanwhile, the national group continued to meet, with England Cancer Czar Mike Richards generally attending each meeting. By now (2006), the government was intent on reducing waiting times for cancer patients, which in turn influenced the star ratings of hospitals and PCTs. This prompted the group to shift its focus from sharing and learning to 'delivering results'. It also started to manage its own meetings.

Against this background, Lisa Godfrey shifted away from facilitation towards more of a management role. Among a variety of approaches to waiting-time reduction, 28 'demonstrator sites' were identified across England – hospitals that had already achieved good results – and Lisa engaged directly with NHS Trust boards to improve performance countrywide. The hospitals were able to make use of a 'how-to guide' that drew on the knowledge and experience of the SIL community, including case studies and top tips for improving cancer waits. Meanwhile, Lisa made sure that she stayed connected with developments 'on the ground' by working on service improvement one day a week in different parts of the NHS.

Lisa described her role with both the national and London groups of SILs as 'one of them, but not a peer'. By 'not a peer', she was making the point that she had access to people and resources that they would not have had without her. Her story demonstrates particularly the possibility of someone moving between community facilitator, budget holder and programme manager as needs change.

## THE VALUE OF SEPARATE AND SKILLED ADMINISTRATORS

Many community facilitators we have spoken with have emphasised the time needed to develop a thriving community. Although the role is not typically full time, one view was that the commitment requires at least 25% of a working week. This means that, if the facilitator has to deal with a lot of administrative problems, they hardly have time left to do the other things that they are there to do. There is therefore generally a strong case for an additional support role. A community administrator can organise the logistics of meetings, process expense claims, write meeting notes, update community information, send out newsletters, track progress of initiatives, and perform a host of other useful (and time-consuming) duties. This frees up the facilitator to focus on developing the community, as we will see in the following story.

### Removing the hassles: the story of a skilled administrator

Lizzie Smith (name changed as the person in question had left Macmillan by the time we wrote this book) was the community administrator for several groups, including the Macmillan GP community and the patient and carer group that worked with it. Lizzie's role was primarily to organise community events and meetings, send out agendas, write up meeting reports and handle expenses and other accounting matters. The GP community was a group of 120 people at the time, so organising the twice-yearly conferences was a much greater task than, for example, running meetings for a group of 15 patients and carers. Lizzie explained:

> *Just keeping the distribution list of the GP Facilitators up to date is a huge challenge. Getting hold of people can be a real administrative nightmare, such as when they don't get back to you about whether or not they are attending a conference. But these things really matter as otherwise people can think that Macmillan has 'forgotten' them. (Lizzie Smith)*

Planning for the GP conferences started several months ahead. The invitation was often tailored for various groups within the community (the engaged, the potentially interested and the more out-of-touch members). The wording was chosen to encourage people to come and, where relevant, to show that Macmillan had noticed that they were absent from previous events. The conferences were a chance to share ideas and experiences and be re-inspired, so it was important to motivate busy people to be there.

At the end of every conference, feedback was gathered from each participant – Lizzie often stood at the door to make sure the forms were handed in, and later she would collate and summarise the comments. These were taken seriously by Macmillan and acted upon for future events.

Lizzie attended all events for her communities. In the case of the GP conferences, this was a busy role over a two-day period – setting up, running around during the event and liaising with hotel staff. Despite the pressure, Lizzie enjoyed this aspect of her role, feeling that she was making an important contribution and was at the centre of things.

With the smaller groups that she supported, Lizzie saw her role as involving more personal relationship building. This was especially true for the patient and carer group, where empathy was important. She was also aware that, for the patients and carers, it was especially important to handle meeting expenses efficiently, if possible reimbursing them with petty cash on the day. This made it as easy as possible for people to participate in the meetings. To support this group well, she felt she needed a combination of efficiency and approachability.

The most difficult aspect of her role, she said, was writing meeting reports. She needed to understand the terminology used in a medical community, despite not being a health professional herself. This was often difficult to follow and the report writing was time consuming, with several editing rounds.

Overall, Lizzie enjoyed this skilled admin role, which she saw as different from working on a normal project:

> *Community events are fun, you feel involved and you get to meet interesting people. Everyone knows who you are and there is always something going on. It is very different to supporting a project where there is a clear start and end date. You get to know community members, you understand what they do and you know who they are as people. (Lizzie Smith)*

As with the community facilitator, the administrator is not generally a full-time role, but it can be an interesting addition to a person's other responsibilities. The key is to select someone with the personal qualities that work well for community support – such as good interpersonal skills, excellent planning and organising skills, an outgoing nature, plenty of initiative and a confident approach to their work.

## ORGANISATIONAL SPONSOR: KEEPING THE SHOW ON THE ROAD

What we mean by the term 'organisational sponsor', in a nutshell, is a manager who acts as the champion for the community, finding necessary resources and helping to ensure that the community connects with the funding organisation. It is important for sponsors to be linked into (or preferably be part of) senior management, as they need to have the authority to dedicate resources to the community. They can also help to engage middle managers, who are particularly likely to feel threatened by the existence of a community that involves their staff, crosses boundaries and cannot be managed like a team or project. Over time we have come to view the organisational sponsor as a challenging but vital role, responsible not only for helping to build effective communities of influence but also for driving programmes of work that emerge from the conversations within communities.

Cultivating communities of influence requires those responsible to 'play a long game'. If the supporting team and community members work well together, results may continue flowing for years to come. However, it can prove difficult to keep other senior managers interested over such long time periods – they may be focused on short-term priorities, or they may get embroiled in restructuring, cost cutting, strategic planning or other typical organisational activities. Moreover, communities of influence are usually invisible on the organisation chart and can seem vague and ephemeral to managers, who may struggle to understand what they actually do and what the 'outcomes' are. All of these factors make the connecting and championing role of organisation sponsor (and community facilitator) vital to a community's survival.

In order to deepen understanding of this role and capture lessons learned in recent years, we invited Glyn Purland, Macmillan's most experienced organisational sponsor (now retired), to talk about his experiences. Our conversation with him brought out a number of themes, which we explore next.

### Satisfying multiple stakeholders

Glyn summarised his own role as follows: 'the organisational sponsor ensures that the outputs from working with a community advance the strategic aims of the organisation'. He went on to distinguish a number of stakeholders and arenas that were relevant to his sponsorship role.

#### Negotiating with senior management

First, he saw himself as having an ongoing responsibility to keep the somewhat fluid conversations and activities of a community in line with what was important to management of the funding organisation. As we have recognised elsewhere, this poses particular challenges, as the people involved in Macmillan communities are generally not its employees. Some were healthcare professionals employed by the

NHS; others were lay people (patients or carers). The relationship between the community and Macmillan was therefore not one of direct authority but rather one of influence and negotiation.

### Orchestrating partnership programmes

Often the programmes and communities sponsored by Glyn involved partnering with policy units in the UK Department of Health, and were therefore referred to as 'partnership programmes'. The need to collaborate with a government department added further layers of complexity to his role. Fortunately, Glyn had worked for many years as a senior manager in the NHS, so he knew his way around it and was used to communicating and negotiating with civil servants. Like the community facilitators described above, he needed to be good at translating and reframing messages for different people.

### Working closely with other members of a supporting team

Glyn recognised the value of the community facilitator role and the need for a strong relationship between sponsor and facilitator. He felt that it was simplest and most effective for the community facilitator (generally a Macmillan employee) to be directly responsible to, and managed by, the sponsor. He also pointed out that, for each of the major initiatives he sponsored, there was a 'clinical lead' (sometimes this was one of the Macmillan GPs) and his relationship with this individual was very important (more about the clinical lead role later in this chapter).

Below we give examples of Glyn's organisational sponsor role in relation to two particular communities: (i) MacPaCC (the group of clinician researchers portrayed in Chapter 5); and (ii) the Macmillan Support Programme for the PCCL (Primary Care Cancer Lead) community described in Chapter 3. Both groups were associated with particular programmes of work aimed at improving services for cancer patients and both involved more than one organisation (e.g. NHS, Macmillan and/or universities). So, Glyn was not only community sponsor but also programme manager and organisational mediator. One thing that set the two stories apart was that, in the first, Glyn was able to pass his sponsorship on to a successor quite smoothly, but in the second this proved more problematic, as we shall see.

## Example 1: sponsoring a group of 'hybrid creatures'

As we saw in Chapter 5, MacPaCC was created to test whether there was value in bringing together clinician researchers, service developers and service users to help improve the care given to people affected by cancer. This particular group had two Macmillan senior managers involved from the beginning. Glyn Purland was one, and the other was head of research Jim Elliott.

Jim took part in MacPaCC meetings and stayed in touch with members between meetings. In addition, as Macmillan's head of research, he played a pivotal part in setting up an innovative and transparent commissioning process and negotiating with group members. This was important because community members were given the opportunity to bid for money intended to pay for research that would help improve the quality of supportive care.

It was Glyn, however, who held the budget for both the research grants and the community (admin support, meetings, etc.). In Glyn's words: 'Authority came not because I could order people around but because I had an overview of what was happening at Macmillan and direct control over financial resources.'

### More than holder of purse strings

Like Jim, Glyn was involved in the negotiations around project funding, but he also contributed in many other ways, including working with clinical leads, helping to articulate the group's purpose (a process that went on for some time) and inviting selected Macmillan managers to community meetings. Together with Jane Maher and Jim Elliott, mentioned earlier, Glyn invited a number of Macmillan senior managers to join the community meetings at different times, so they could see members in action, benefit from their knowledge and experience and also share developments in Macmillan's strategic thinking.

### A smooth handover

Glyn noted that, as he took on other major programmes, it became increasingly difficult for him to give MacPaCC the political support it needed. At a time when Macmillan was going through a turbulent period of review and restructuring, he found himself less and less at the heart of general policymaking in the charity. Jane Maher was able to make a successful case for continuing support for the group to a new senior budget holder (Macmillan's new head of research). The tangible research results from this group (all logged as part of the narrative tracking) played an important part in convincing the funders of its ongoing value. After 2007, MacPaCC went from strength to strength with a new organisational sponsor in place.

The MacPaCC story throws up a number of lessons about community sponsorship, including:

- authority derives from being the budget holder, even when the sponsor does not have direct management control of the members of the group
- it is important to *negotiate* the group's 'direction of travel' or 'terms of reference', rather than trying to impose them
- restructuring in the funding organisation can cause disruption, potentially making it harder for the sponsor to continue acting as a bridge between the community and its funder

- other members of the supporting team can provide continuity if and when the organisational sponsor needs to hand over responsibility.

**Example 2: 'inspiration and perspiration' – the PCCL community**

In the second example of Glyn's sponsorship role, we return to the PCCLs referred to in Chapter 3. There we saw how Macmillan chose to support the development of this community, without actually funding the health professionals' protected time (that was the responsibility of the NHS). The Macmillan Support Programme, as it was known, committed £3 million over five years to developing a sizeable community of lead clinicians. Glyn acted as a highly visible sponsor and 'Macmillan voice' for this comprehensive programme of support and professional development, working in partnership with consultancy Innové.

It is notable that both community and programme had emerged partly from discussions among Macmillan GP Advisors. However, it needed a senior manager to build on what the GP Advisors had begun. As Glyn put it, 'The responsibility for making it all happen in detail fell to me as Macmillan manager.'

For about five years from 2001, Glyn worked with Rosie Loftus, who had taken over from another GP Advisor (Greg Tanner) as clinical lead for the PCCL community. As the programme drew to a close in 2006, Glyn summed up his experience as community (and programme) sponsor in a way that clearly brings out two key aspects – being able both to work with clinical leaders and to 'translate' the value of the community to senior policymakers:

> *The project has been a success and the PCCL role is now embedded in the NHS. This is thanks to inspiration from Greg and some perspiration from me. I have always been totally comfortable with this. It is important having people who can take sparks/ideas, and can 'earth the glitter-brains' – and in any case, doctors are only involved part time. I fronted the relationship with the Department of Health (funding, planning, approvals, etc.) and this freed up Greg and later Rosie to think primarily as clinicians. They could safely be 'dogmatic' about the project because they knew I could re-present what they said for Department of Health ears. (Glyn Purland)*

As the Macmillan Support Programme was nearing its scheduled end in 2006, Macmillan set up a second 'distilling-and-connecting' group (known as the PCCL Forum) along the lines of the GP Advisor group, in order to maintain the connection between Macmillan and the widely dispersed PCCLs. This distilling-and-connecting group (like the GPA group described in Chapter 3) was much more compact than the community it served, so it could develop a close working relationship with the supporting team. The idea was that it would be a community of influence in its own right. Glyn acted as organisational sponsor for the PCCL Forum until his retirement in 2007, when Macmillan funding for this group was discontinued.

We put down the limited life of this particular distilling-and-connecting group to a combination of factors. First, Glyn began to reduce his workload with Macmillan in 2006–07, so sponsorship of the Forum was handed over to a new Macmillan sponsor just a few months after the group was created. She took part in what turned out to be the community's last two meetings but she did not have a history of working with the Macmillan communities of influence and had no prior involvement with the PCCLs as a group, so she was more of a 'caretaker' than a committed sponsor. Second, there was no community facilitator (Lorraine Sloan having moved into another role inside Macmillan). And third, clinical lead Rosie Loftus proposed that the Macmillan GP Advisors could act as the distilling-and-connecting group for the PCCL community, a role they already performed for the Macmillan GPs. This meant that in the view of the new sponsor and the clinical lead, there was no longer a rationale for the PCCL Forum to continue as a separate community.

From the experience of setting up the PCCL Forum, it is clear that different organisational sponsors will have different views on how best to maintain the connection between community and funding organisation.

**Tips for potential sponsors**

Glyn offered the following suggestions to anyone taking on an organisational sponsorship role for the first time.

- Stay close to the funding organisation's strategic aims – preferably be part of developing them.
- Keep direct control of all relevant budgets.
- Be prepared to stay with the community or programme for three to five years; it takes at least 18 months to build relationships, and the longer a group works together the more effective it can become.
- Only take on the role if you feel personally committed to the aims of the group/community; sponsorship is more than just a piece of work to be done, it's about real commitment and championing.
- Take time to understand and get comfortable with the other senior people working with the group and decide how to play your role in relation to theirs.

Glyn's background as a senior NHS manager over a number of years helped him to be very comfortable with the sponsor role. He was used to influencing people over whom he had little or no line authority, building consensus, thinking strategically, behaving collaboratively, as well as designing and delivering cross-boundary healthcare programmes. He felt that the role should be recognised in a number of contexts – communities, programmes, campaigns – and that the right people should be positioned in the role with enough continuity and support to ensure that investments are realised and lessons learned.

We have seen that it requires a special kind of senior manager to work with clinicians and make things happen. The individual may have a dual role as both sponsor for the community and manager of any programmes associated with that community. In the final stages of a time-limited programme (like the Macmillan Support Programme for the PCCLs), the sponsoring organisation needs to think hard about whether the community merits continued support and investment, or whether it should be wound down because a work programme is complete. We have become increasingly convinced that there is a strong case for sustaining a community of influence after such a programme has concluded. The ongoing relationships and conversations can enable the funding organisation to continue getting value out of its investment.

## DISTILLING-AND-CONNECTING GROUPS

As we have seen, a distilling-and-connecting group is a community within a community. The first one mentioned in this book was the Macmillan GP Advisor group (*see* Chapter 3). The purpose of this selected group of active community members was to 'distil' the experiences and views of the wider GP community and connect it to other movers and shakers.

The advantage of having a distilling-and-connecting group is that a few enthusiastic community members can have a hand in steering the community, taking up ideas and doing some of the vital connecting or political work. Having such a group also gives the sponsor and facilitator more people to call on to help with events, projects, meetings with policymakers, and any other community-related issues.

The distilling-and-connecting group is an interesting variation on the more traditional 'steering group' or 'advisory group' often set up for programmes of work. Both go beyond just consulting members on specific issues. However, what is different about a distilling-and-connecting group, in our experience, is that it can act as a 'living link' between a larger community of influence and the funder(s).

If the larger community of influence has a clinical lead (Rosie Loftus in the case of the Macmillan GP community – *see* portrait below), then that person will probably be part of the distilling-and-connecting group. They add a different perspective to that of the community sponsor, whose primary concern has to be the needs of the sponsoring organisation or organisations. The clinical lead is also often in a good position to suggest members for the distilling-and-connecting group.

For practical purposes it is probably best to keep a distilling-and-connecting group to a manageable size, say up to about 12 people, as this can make it much easier to agree a direction of travel and to deepen relationships. In the way that Macmillan has developed it, the distilling-and-connecting group can also be viewed as a community of influence in its own right. The way members are selected is therefore different from normal committees or working groups. Macmillan has tried a number of approaches in setting up such groups – conducting a democratic nomination process with the wider community, identifying the most willing and enthusiastic volunteers, or 'cherry picking' specific individuals based on their collaborative spirit, their experience, and the respect of their peers ('he/she is one of us'). Although no method is perfect, in our experience the latter approach is most likely to ensure the group is productive and influential.

Each GP Advisor developed their role to make the most of their own talents and interests.

## PORTRAIT OF ROSIE LOFTUS, MACMILLAN GP ADVISOR

Rosie's background included 15 years working as a GP and four years in a hospice. Her formal connection with Macmillan began in 2001 when she started a three-year stint as a Macmillan GP (GP Facilitator).

Macmillan offered her the post of GP Advisor in 2002, to be linked into the charity's regional team in southeast England. The role appealed to her in more ways than one: she appreciated the need to support the Macmillan GPs in her region (she had been one herself), and also she could see how hard it was to spread good ideas.

### Living link

Rosie's work as a GP Advisor had a number of strands: (i) developing initiatives in primary care (service development); (ii) participating in national activities in pursuit of better cancer care; and (iii) 'pastoral' work, which involved recruiting and supporting Macmillan GPs in her region – their number grew from six to 24. It was this last strand that most interested her, so she chose to focus particularly on supporting and linking the GPs. For example, she regularly participated in the two-monthly meetings of the northeast London group of Macmillan GPs. She also tried setting up an online discussion facility after many requests for a website but, interestingly, found that it was little used.

Being an Advisor meant working closely with Macmillan's regional team, which included five Service Development Managers (SDMs). Each SDM was quite different. For example, one had had vast experience of working with Macmillan GPs, while another had none, so Rosie's involvement varied to match their wants. Since the SDMs had administrative and contract responsibility for the Macmillan GPs, Rosie always tried to speak to the relevant SDM before she met the GP in question. She particularly liked to sort out any issues that arose (e.g. about payment of protected time) quickly. And if someone expressed an interest in becoming a Macmillan GP, she made sure they got a quick response too.

Looking after the Macmillan GPs, though satisfying, presented Rosie with challenges. For example, when she asked them for an annual report in order to capture some of the lessons learned from the work, only three in ten supplied it. In addition, she would have liked to appraise the GPs but could not because she was not their line manager. Finally, sometimes it was hard to work out who was good at the role, because if someone wasn't effective (which was rare) it might have something to do with the context (e.g. relationship with their local NHS organisation).

### A birthday party with a serious point

One particular anecdote demonstrates Rosie's talent for bringing people together. At a Macmillan national GP conference near Northampton in June 2004, she ran a meeting for the Macmillan GPs from her region as a 'birthday party', having discovered previously that one of the GPs actually had a birthday on the day. She handed round a large bag overflowing with colourfully wrapped presents, asking each participant to unwrap a parcel as well as telling the group about one happy or exciting incident that had happened to them in the past year. The parcels contained useful booklets (e.g. on benefits), information sheets (e.g. on 'enhanced services') or forms (e.g. the surgery bereavement form), and Rosie picked someone in the room who could explain what each item was, how it came to be, how you might use it, etc. This enabled her to draw people's attention to the wide range of materials available to Macmillan GPs, while also stimulating storytelling and learning within the group. At the end of the workshop, every participant received the whole set of documents to take home.

### Burning midnight oil

By 2004, Rosie's working life had myriad elements. When we spoke to her, her working week included two days in her GP practice, two days as a GP Advisor, half a day as a PCCL, and half a day working on the GSF. She enjoyed all these roles, and found that they allowed her to use the valuable skills associated with being a GP, e.g. facilitation and negotiation. Nonetheless, it was a demanding week for a working parent: 'In every part-time role, people assume you work full time. . . . The problem is that the emails never stop coming . . . but then two hours spent emailing after the children are in bed is no worse than two hours of TV'.

As someone who gave so much to supporting others, where did Rosie get her own support? The immediate answer was her family. But also, being a member of the GP Advisor group helped her feel she was not 'a bod in the wilderness'. For example, early on in her role as GP Advisor, a GP complained that Rosie was less available than her predecessor, though he couldn't give any examples of this problem. Rosie rang experienced GP Advisor David Millar, explained the situation and asked him if he thought she was doing anything wrong. From his experience, he was able to reassure her that she was not.

As Macmillan's Lead GP Advisor, Rosie was (and still is) both a member of the distilling-and-connecting group for the charity's GP community and a clinical lead. It is the clinical lead role that we look at next – what is special about it and what skills and personal qualities does it demand?

## CLINICAL LEADER: SKILLED TRANSLATOR AND INFLUENCER

In a sense, all members of the Macmillan-sponsored communities of influence are leaders, whether locally or nationally. But often one particular individual emerges from within the membership and begins to act as 'the face' of the community. For example, after some time as a member of the GPA group, Rosie Loftus became 'Macmillan Lead GP Advisor'. This made her the clinical lead for the whole Macmillan GP community and she was also instrumental in expanding the capacity of the GPA team. Compared with the five members in the early 2000s, by 2010 this was a distilling-and-connecting group with 15 members.

### Knowing what it's like to live in a clinician's world

So, what does a clinical lead like Rosie Loftus bring to the table? First, by continuing to be rooted in a general practice, she knows what it is like to live in a clinician's world and has credibility among 'jobbing GPs'. This means she can interpret back and forth between GPs, the sponsoring organisation and senior figures in the NHS. For example, she can translate managerial language into GP-speak, and vice versa. As well as speaking the language of GPs and helping to make the community and its initiatives more visible to management, the clinical leader can also initiate or take part in high-level meetings with senior decision-makers or government representatives.

### A clinical partner for community facilitator and organisational sponsor

We found that, in the best cases, the clinical leader became a much-valued partner to both community facilitator and organisational sponsor. When all three work together, they can ensure that the work of the community of influence is well connected with the sponsoring organisation and other stakeholders.

What makes this kind of partnership work? Obviously it helps if these individuals get on well together. Another aspect mentioned by Lorraine Sloan who, as we have seen, increasingly found herself managing the programmes of work that emerged from the GP community, was that she and Rosie could go to high-level meetings as a duo. Both Lorraine and Rosie felt that acting in partnership like this was helpful. A clinical lead without a manager or sponsor from the funding organisation might not get the support needed to pursue large-scale change. But equally, a programme manager without a clinical lead might give clinicians the impression that the funding organisation wants to tell them what to do.

Another contribution that Rosie Loftus made was her willingness to share her contacts with Lorraine and Macmillan. For example, she had existing relationships with a key technology provider for GP information systems. This helped ensure that general practices recorded precisely what they covered when they reviewed a cancer patient's needs and care.

From the organisational sponsor's point of view, the clinical lead may be the one clinician they speak to regularly. The partnership works best if it is an equal one, even though holding the purse strings may seem to give the organisational sponsor a slight edge.

### What qualities and skills does a clinical lead need?

Rosie indicated some of the skills needed to be a good clinical lead for a community of influence:

- tolerance and patience – it takes patience to work with bureaucratic processes
- influencing and negotiating skills
- being well connected
- willingness and qualities needed to be 'the face of the community' and not 'say the wrong thing'
- ability to wear multiple hats, depending, for example, on whether talking to clinicians or senior directors.

The last point echoes our notion of 'hybrid creatures' (*see* Chapter 5) – like them, the clinical leader can wear many different hats and needs to have credibility with a number of different stakeholders, such as clinicians, service developers, managers, policymakers and researchers.

Finally, when asked what she had learned from her experience of the lead role, Rosie said she had come to understand organisation culture better and to work with it, which required pragmatism and patience at times. The one piece of advice she offered to others was: 'If you think a project is worth doing, stick with it'. She went on to explain why GPs might sometimes find this kind of work frustrating:

> *GPs can be task-orientated – they see a patient, diagnose and treat them. So they can see their impact. In GP-land, you want to make a difference and you see what*

*happens. But as a clinical leader, you don't always know what difference you have made. The good thing about it, though, is that it enables you to reach more people. (Rosie Loftus)*

## POINTS TO CONSIDER WHEN CULTIVATING COMMUNITIES OF INFLUENCE

Below we have distilled some general points to guide those considering setting up a community of influence, whether it is a sizeable network of professionals, a 'distilling-and-connecting group', or a group of service users (e.g. patients and/or carers).

### Choosing members

When building a community of influence, the choice of members is critical and their potential reach and influence needs to be a major criterion for membership. It is not always obvious who is – or should be – in a community of influence. Is it for anyone who expresses an interest in joining? Is it just the 'movers and shakers'? Is it only for people of a certain seniority? Is it a global or national community, or only for certain localities? The best ideas often come from groups that include people with different perspectives and access to a wide range of personal networks.

Ideally, community sponsor, community facilitator and clinical lead (if there is one) work together with a few of the community members to agree both criteria and process. Potential new members may then be identified by any of the above. Once members have been suggested, the community sponsor and/or the distilling-and-connecting group may want to review them. If they are accepted, the formal invitation can come from the community sponsor and/or clinical lead, with the community facilitator contacting the new member to welcome them personally into the group. The process tends to be fluid and relationship-based rather than bureaucratic – unlike the typical membership structures in more traditional clubs or associations.

It may sound obvious, but it is important to know who the members are, so that clear communication can be established with them – and also so that other interested individuals understand why they are *not* included in the community processes. As a rule we find it is best to be inclusive rather than exclusive – it is possible to communicate cost effectively with a broad group of people. A 'cost-benefit calculation' can then be made to decide who can be invited to face-to-face events, since these tend to be the biggest investment of time and money. Invitations to events should make it clear what the criteria for inclusion are, e.g. first-come-first-served, nominations, interest in the topics covered at the event, relevant experience and/or level of seniority.

Many communities find themselves with three types of members.

- *Core members:* Most communities of influence have a core of committed and active members who fully participate in all community activities (this is a perfectly natural aspect of larger groups)
- *An extended list of people:* Included in the community's communication processes but might only be invited to face-to-face events as special guests for a specific reason
- *Stakeholders:* People interested in the community's activities who may be occasional guests at community events but are not members of the community per se. In the Macmillan context, these might be Department of Health policy people, for example.

### Handling 'exits' with care

It is worth considering whether membership should be time limited (perhaps two or three years), so that fresh perspectives can be regularly brought into the group. As mentioned, community members contribute their time voluntarily and there may come a time when they are ready to move on for any number of reasons. This need not be viewed as a problem, provided their 'exit' is handled well. Community facilitator, sponsor and lead clinician can all play a part in showing that the individual's contribution has been acknowledged and appreciated. The person's relationship with remaining members and sponsoring organisations may well continue to generate influence and service improvements for years to come.

### Scheduling planning and reflection time for the supporting team

As soon as the decision has been made to create a community, the community sponsor, facilitator and clinical lead (the 'supporting team') may wish to plan a regular series of phone calls or meetings to prepare the ground. Frequency for community meetings is worth agreeing on early, and the dates noted in people's diaries well in advance. It will then be important for the supporting team to meet a few weeks or even months in advance of each community event so that they can do all the necessary preparation in good time. Some or all of these conversations can include the distilling-and-connecting group, if one has been established.

After a community meeting it is always valuable for the supporting team to get together to reflect on how it went and what else needs doing. If team members need to race off immediately after a community meeting, e.g. to catch a train or plane, a separate 'debrief' meeting is worth scheduling.

With Macmillan communities, we scheduled all the meetings of the supporting team up to a whole year in advance. Without proper preparation and reflection, a promising community can wither on the vine due to lack of time and attention.

### Negotiating a 'direction of travel' with the community

Different communities develop according to different patterns. For example, the Macmillan GP community first introduced in Chapter 1 started as a pilot scheme with just six GP Facilitators and later grew into a community of 100 members and more. In contrast, the clinician researcher group described in Chapter 5 never grew larger than about a dozen regular members – it was created for quite a different purpose, namely to produce evidence needed to improve care for dying cancer patients and also form a collaborative research group.

No matter which chain of events leads to the birth of the community, it is important to think about how to encourage members to have the conversations needed to develop a common sense of purpose. Thus, in the early days of a community's existence, one of the most important conversations is one in which members and supporting team jointly explore and clarify the community's aims and priorities. We have found that this can take considerable time. Indeed, it may continue throughout the life of the community. This 'iterative' process can be new to people who are used to a funding organisation telling them what to do. But the end result is more likely to be a group committed to achieving outcomes they helped to shape rather than reluctantly conforming to someone else's agenda.

It can be beneficial to document the outcome from these conversations, creating a kind of 'community charter' (sometimes more conventionally known as 'terms of reference'), which may be reviewed and amended over time. The process of creating such a charter can help to develop everybody's thinking, and the document produced will also be helpful to new members or other people with an interest in the community.

### Creating conditions for productive community meetings

The face-to-face meetings of communities of influence are the most visible investments of time, money and energy for all concerned, and it is these live encounters that determine the community's success more than anything else. We have found that regular face-to-face meetings allow trusting relationships to develop, experiences to be shared and conversations to spark action. The very act of coming together – to talk and work out what could be achieved collectively – is vital. It therefore pays to think carefully about how to invite people to join, set the tone of meetings, encourage collaborative working from the start and create community meetings that are conducive to sharing knowledge, developing a collective voice and expanding people's influencing capacities.

If these community gatherings are treated like standard business meetings, they are unlikely to be either productive or energising (just as many business meetings prove to be a waste of time). There is a real skill to designing lively and useful community meetings, and it may be worth engaging an experienced consultant or 'convenor' (we use this term in order to distinguish this person from the community facilitator) to co-design and run the meetings, particularly if this is not one of the skills of the community facilitator. (With the Macmillan communities, the convenor, like the narrative writer, was typically an external consultant.)

In the box below are some tips for designing community events, based on experience across a range of organisational settings. There are many small things that can make a big difference when a community meets.

### Making meetings both welcoming and productive

Designing an effective community event requires skill and experience. It is not a traditional task-focused meeting but an opportunity to learn and build relationships. If the community sponsor and facilitators are not experienced in designing this type of event, it is advisable to get help from someone who is highly skilled at 'convening'.

Health professionals and managers can be very task-focused, so investing time and energy in building a foundation of personal relationships and trust can be a new experience for them. It may feel like a waste of time when in fact it is one of the most essential aspects of building a strong community. It's simple: if you build trust, effective collaboration will follow. If you don't, it won't.

#### *First meeting*

The first meeting of a community is critical as it sets the tone for how members will work together. It is also the first opportunity to start building working relationships that may last for years. It is advisable, where possible, to make this a residential event with at least one overnight stay, to give people the opportunity to socialise together.

To set a collaborative tone and encourage networking, people will need time to get to know each other. This is an essential part of building trust and goodwill. As most people know, times spent talking informally in a bar or restaurant are often the most productive conversations of all. If it is possible to hold the meeting as a residential event, it is often useful to start with dinner one evening, keep formal 'input' to a minimum and simply give people an opportunity to get to know each other. This is an additional cost but there is a long-term return on the investment. By the time discussions start the following morning, you will have a group of people who know something about each other and are ready to move into productive work. This also reduces the risk of people arriving late and missing the important stage of personal introductions.

When a community first meets, it can be helpful to invite people to say something about their interests outside of work. In our experience, this can completely shift the tone of the meeting. It helps people to come out from behind their organisational façades and appear as human beings.

### *Introductions*

Even if people already know each other, there may be merit in scheduling some social time before the formal start of community meetings. Moreover, any new members or guests can be introduced informally at this point. It may also be a good idea, even if people have been introduced, to give everyone a chance to speak at the official start of the community meeting. One way of doing this is to ask participants what their hopes and fears are regarding the community. This gives them permission to open up and talk about their feelings. It also values and recognises every individual in the room and brings out some things to foster (or avoid) in future.

### *Negotiating the agenda*

People who treat a community event like any other meeting may make the mistake of applying a traditional meeting structure to it. In other words, someone determines the agenda, fills every minute with items, and perhaps even structures it around Powerpoint presentations, leaving little time for discussion. This may result in some information being shared but it will do little to build trust, share knowledge or encourage collaboration. We think a different approach is needed. First, any formal agenda, if required, should be proposed and discussed with community members before being agreed. Second, the event should have plenty of 'open space' for dialogue. The social time will provide some of that but the meeting structure should also allow for open discussion. It is unlikely that a community meeting should be any shorter than a full day and, in view of earlier comments about social time, at least a day and a half is preferable.

In our experience it helps to accept that many people are accustomed to focusing on tasks or projects (and often worried that nothing will come of a meeting where people apparently 'just talk'). One way of easing their concerns is to provide enough 'structure' or 'content' in the early part of the community meeting, e.g. by inviting a guest to give a short talk, or allowing time for members to work in small groups on specific projects or issues. With a sense of having done something 'productive', people seem to have more appetite to spend time in more reflective mode, e.g. sharing experiences or stories that help the group to reach a deeper understanding of the nature of 'collaborative influence'.

### *Physical working environment*

The physical environment can make a huge difference to how a group feels about working together. If you want a community to get off to a bad start, book your first meeting in a cramped airless room with no windows and provide standard sandwiches as the lunchtime fare. If you want to increase its chances of success, book a venue away from people's offices, provide an airy, spacious room with lots of natural light and make sure the catering is good. This doesn't necessarily mean spending lots of money. However it is a false economy to skimp on the budget for community events and put people into an environment that they can't wait to escape from. A pleasant working environment is one way to say that this community is important and its members are valued. This is one area where charitable organisations may look to commercial sponsors such as pharmaceutical companies to pay for a good venue, as long as the sponsor does not alter the spirit of the meetings in some undesirable way or use them for their own ends.

#### *Seating arrangements*

Linked to the physical working environment is the question of how people are seated in the room. Of course this will depend on the numbers involved and the way the room is furnished, but the key design principle should be openness and equality of status. A collection of small (ideally round) tables arranged 'café style' around the room encourages interaction. Another option is to have people seated in a circle (or semicircle if somebody is giving a talk) without any tables at all. Having no physical barriers contributes to relationship building. If there are presentations, ensure everyone can see well and is close enough to engage in dialogue.

#### *People arriving late or leaving early*

People who arrive late for an event – whatever the reason may be and even if it is only by a quarter of an hour – may be seen by others as less committed to the community. That first negative impression will be set and may take some time to be readjusted. Leaving early will have the same effect. It is therefore important to encourage everyone to be there for the whole event.

### Nurturing the community between meetings

Face-to-face meetings inject energy into a community. People often leave such meetings filled with enthusiasm and committed to taking action. However it is a sad reality that day-to-day life intervenes and often drains that energy away. Back-to-back work meetings, dealing with endless emails and phone calls, the pressure of other work priorities – all of these conspire to sap the energy of community members. Community sponsors and facilitators – especially the latter – have a key role to play to keep the community energy flowing between meetings. The vital ingredient is the energy and care of the facilitators themselves; they can keep people in touch by communicating with them and sharing relevant and useful information. (If an external convenor and narrative writer are engaged, they too may make a point of staying in touch with community members between meetings.)

Regular communication can also help to make community members feel valued and appreciated. For example, if a member has led a discussion or given a presentation at a community event, a personal telephone call to thank them will show appreciation and encourage future contributions. These kinds of regular communications are a vital aspect of community building that Wenger, *et al.* have called the 'heartbeat of the community'.[2]

### Using technology (with caution)

In the 21st century, information technology can connect groups of people across time and distance. Regular email communication, telephone or video conferences, newsletters and online discussion forums are all options for keeping contact between community members. Community facilitators need to consider which methods will work best for their community. Although they involve time and effort they can save the time of community members by giving them easy access to important knowledge and information.

It is very likely that there will be a case for creating a 'virtual online home' for the community, not only as a place to share information cost-effectively but also as a means of reinforcing the community's sense of identity. Finding a community member (or other person) with the interest and skill to set up the community's virtual home is an early and valuable task for the community facilitator. Many software products are available for this purpose, including free ones such as Google sites, Yahoo groups or Facebook groups. In our experience one should not expect too much of such tools. Most communities make use of only a few core features, typically including a repository of shared information (communities sometimes use 'wiki' technology for this purpose) and a 'Who's Who' of community members with photos and contact details. Some people will want a discussion forum to enable them to see and contribute to exchanges without clogging their email inboxes.

It is arguable that any influential professional network or think tank *must* have a web presence nowadays, so that people beyond the group can find out who is in it, what it stands for, what it has accomplished and what it is pursuing. A dedicated website can provide health professionals, researchers, educators, policymakers, managers and others with succinct information about the group and its achievements – it is indispensable for any serious community of influence that wants to have a voice in its field. The use of technology is about making the community and its work visible. It complements but is distinct from the collaborative tools described above.

### Assembling a supporting team

In this chapter, we have described the kind of supporting team needed to develop a thriving community of influence. To recap, below is a summary of key roles. The first three people on the list will most likely be employees of the sponsoring organisation, the others not.

- An organisational sponsor who acts as the champion for the

community, finds the necessary resources and keeps it linked to the strategic aims of the funding organisation.
- A facilitator (or facilitators) who provides continuity and keeps the community both energised and focused.
- A separate administrative person to organise meetings, maintain information resources, etc.
- In the healthcare sector, there may be a case for working with a clinical lead who speaks the language of whichever group of professionals makes up the community and can help shape the group's priorities.
- If the community is large, it may be worth considering creating a smaller group (a 'community within a community') that will work closely with the funding organisation, to distil learning from community conversations and act as a living link between community, funding organisation and the wider world.
- Finally, there may be benefit in engaging external consultants/writers to convene community meetings and write the narrative accounts, if the considerable skills needed for these roles are not available in-house.

### Establishing a budget

Communities of influence need investment if they are to succeed. One key element in the healthcare sector is funding for 'protected time', also sometimes referred to as 'backfill'. This enables professionals to participate in community activities by ensuring that their clinical role is covered for that period of time. For example, Macmillan often provides GPs or nurses with protected time by paying backfill costs (typically for the first three years in post), to enable them to work in partnership with the organisation and participate in community events.

The salaries of the supporting team are usually paid either by the sponsoring organisation(s) or by their employer (e.g. the NHS). In addition it is likely that a budget will be required to cover the expenses of the group – paying travel costs, for example, can make the difference between a group being able to meet or not.

Our experience with Macmillan and other organisations has revealed a number of funding models, for example, a central budget provided by one or more sponsoring organisations, a subscription model (where members and/or their organisations pay into a central pot to cover community activities), or simply an agreement that members will pay their own expenses. Enabling communities of influence to do real work takes time and money, and additional money may be required to pursue specific projects. The challenge of securing a budget usually falls on the shoulders of the community sponsor(s).

Finally, with any community of influence, it is important to recognise when to draw the funding to a close. This will inevitably reduce connectedness but a few people will probably stay in touch nevertheless.

### Increasing the community's visibility

There is always a danger that the costs of the community (travel expenses, meeting costs, people's time) are more visible than the benefits (good ideas shared, productive conversations, stakeholders influenced). It is therefore important to track a community's evolution and achievements, as we showed in Chapter 2, to help maintain the motivation and enthusiasm of sponsor(s), facilitators and members; if the value of the community remains invisible to the funder(s), it may become impossible to sustain the investment.

The best person to listen out for and note down stories of how the community is making a difference may be the community facilitator, but in our experience it is sometimes crucial to bring in a professional writer who understands the way communities of influence work. Among other things, this person needs to understand that many valuable and unplanned results arise simply by virtue of bringing together a diverse group of committed human beings, and that these unplanned outcomes are part of what is tracked and captured. They add to the evidence needed to demonstrate 'return on investment'.

## PITFALLS TO WATCH OUT FOR

Establishing and nurturing a community of influence is an art more than a science. We have learned over time that there are certain moments in the life of a community when the going may get tough. Below we identify some of these moments and make some suggestions for how best to handle them.

### Changing sponsors and/or facilitators

As described earlier in this chapter, community sponsors and facilitators play key roles in the life of a community. However, these individuals may move on and it is important to plan for their replacement by identifying and preparing possible successors. We have seen examples of successful communities that died a 'sudden death' because key sponsors or facilitators moved on with no ready replacement. The demise of the community is usually not due to lack of interest but, more pragmatically, the lack of a person to organise meetings and communication (facilitation role), or lack of influence in the right places to protect the community (sponsorship role).

In our experience, if the person in any of the three main roles – organisational sponsor, clinical lead, community facilitator – changes or leaves, there is a risk that the community meetings will cease (though some of the relationships formed will almost certainly continue).

When an organisational sponsor or community facilitator moves on it is important to communicate the new arrangements to the group. Otherwise, resentment or confusion can easily build up – if group members are good networkers they can spread negative as well as positive messages.

### Misapprehension about a community's purpose

Another threat to a community's long-term viability and success is lack of clarity of purpose. If stakeholders have expectations that differ from what it produces, it may be seen as unsuccessful, whereas in fact it might simply be working to a different agenda. Confusion typically develops when *tangible* products are expected from a community whose actual goal is to influence fellow professionals and/or decision-makers, or to improve services locally but without a highly visible output. Such mismatch of expectations may threaten community funding, and sponsors and facilitators have an important role in clarifying and communicating the purposes of the community – especially if they change over time.

### 'It's a clique'

When selecting members for a community of influence one pitfall is that people outside the community may perceive it as a collection of someone's cronies. While there are practical reasons for limiting the size of a community, it is best to be transparent about the process by which people are invited to participate.

### Destructive behaviour

Communities can be destroyed from within. In any group of people involved in a common endeavour there will be conflict, subtle or open. A degree of this can be viewed as 'creative tension' and be resolved without difficulty. However, people's behaviour within communities sometimes becomes poisonous, perhaps due to relationship breakdowns with other members of the community, or to a fundamental disagreement with the direction a community is taking. A challenge for sponsors and facilitators is to recognise when a problem has become serious and to deal with it firmly. A quiet one-to-one conversation may be sufficient to influence the person's behaviour, but it may ultimately be necessary to stop inviting them to community events.

### Perceived as a threat to the established order

Communities of influence – organic, non-hierarchical but potentially powerful nonetheless – can be perceived as a threat by the hierarchies that they touch. Members' employers/managers may feel threatened or left out, realising they have no control over what the community is doing. They may even try to sabotage their staff member's involvement, e.g. by refusing to pay expenses or not allowing them to attend community meetings. The community sponsor and facilitator can mitigate this risk by talking to the manager about the community's role and the benefits it aims to deliver, and by encouraging them to support their staff member's involvement.

We hope that by highlighting these pitfalls we are increasing the chances of creating a successful community of influence rather than discouraging anyone from trying.

## NOTES

1 www.collinslanguage.com (23 December 2010).
2 Wenger E, McDermott R, Snyder W. *Cultivating Communities of Practice: a guide to managing knowledge.* Boston, MA: Harvard Business School Press; 2002.

CHAPTER 7

# Involving lay people as partners

## How patients joined a professional community and helped shape new services

### OVERVIEW

*We think of the groups of 'service users' created by Macmillan to influence and shape programmes of work or new services, as communities of influence in their own right. We have already met the patient and carer group that produced* Our Principles of People-Centred Care. *From 2003, members of this group were invited into the meetings of the Macmillan GP community, in order to help it stay grounded in the needs of ordinary patients and carers, and this experience confirmed the importance of preparing people for such encounters. Later on, another group of patients and carers was created specially to inform a national programme whose purpose was to develop services for those with a family history of cancer.*

*Organisations wishing to encourage or sponsor such activities face a choice between different forms of partnership – ranging from small, intensively supported groups to much larger, more inclusive networks of volunteers. What is clear is that people who have had a life-changing experience are often moved to do something to help others who find themselves in a similar predicament. This is highly pertinent for anybody interested in what 'citizen empowerment' might mean in practice.*

As we saw in Chapter 1, insights from early work with patient self-help groups in southeast England provided some of the inspiration for Macmillan's later work with GPs and communities of influence. We resume the patient involvement story in the early 2000s, when Macmillan was intensifying its relationship with doctors and created a group of people living with cancer (including both patients and carers) to advise it specifically on this work.[1] We think of such service-user groups as communities of influence in their own right and, as with all such communities, regular face-to-face meetings are a vital part of their work. One of this particular group's most visible achievements was the poster-sized guide called *Our Principles of People-Centred Care* (*see* Chapter 4).

## INTRODUCING LAY PEOPLE INTO A COMMUNITY OF GPs

Not long after this group's formation, Macmillan began to invite its members into the twice-yearly conferences of its GP community. Bringing patients and carers into a professional community is not a simple task. Patients may not always feel confident in speaking up in front of health professionals and typically there is a perceived power imbalance between patients and doctors. Lorraine Sloan, community facilitator of both communities (GPs and people living with cancer), pointed to some of the challenges she encountered:

> *It was brave of Macmillan to bring user involvement into the GP community. Things got off to a flying start but after a while they took a bit of a dip. I couldn't understand why, so I phoned some of the GPs to find out. They said they felt that we were bringing in people whose stories were not typical of the kind of patients they had seen coming through their doors. They felt that some fresh voices were needed. (Lorraine Sloan)*

Given these concerns, Lorraine and her colleagues started to encourage the people living with cancer to bring new people to the Macmillan-sponsored meetings. The 'old hands' were urged to 'buddy up' with newer people, so the latter could get to grips with their role more quickly.

Another major issue that emerged was that people living with cancer appeared to have a limited understanding of the challenges facing GPs. At the Macmillan GP conference in October 2004, which was attended by patients and carers for the first time, one of the GPs was talking to Lorraine about this. They agreed to put together an 'Ask the GP anything' panel session, in which a GP gave a presentation on 'a morning in my life as a GP', with anonymous details of each patient she saw and her thought process in assessing them. What she was showing was that history, patient examination and findings are all very similar for patients with and without cancer. With many patients, she might think they *could* have cancer, but most of them will turn out *not* to have it. The session was extremely well evaluated: at the start, people were asked about the role of the GP in cancer and most thought it was small; by the end, when views were sought again, attitudes had shifted, and several went on to become champions for the role of GPs in cancer and palliative care. The people living with cancer who attended this session also reported feeling better prepared to work in partnership with GPs.

The 'Ask the GP anything' session lived on and provided much of the thinking that went into an e-learning module that Macmillan created in 2010. This became one of many ways of preparing lay people to take part in professional communities of influence.

## NEW SERVICES FOR PEOPLE WITH A FAMILY HISTORY OF CANCER

The emphasis in the example above was on introducing patients and carers into a community made up mainly of professionals. Next we tell the story of another group of patients and carers that was set up by Macmillan specifically to help establish services across England for people with a family history of cancer. From 2004 to 2007, Macmillan Cancer Support and the Department of Health co-sponsored a programme to explore ways of identifying people at risk and providing them with advice, care and support. The programme involved setting up seven pilot services across England, based in primary and secondary care. The 'Cancer Genetics Pilots Programme', as it was known, gave service-user involvement high priority. As well as sitting on the programme steering group, service users contributed to every pilot project.

Macmillan also gave service users from each pilot project the opportunity to gather four times a year as a national user reference group (NURG). The NURG can be seen as a community of influence, even though its lifespan was limited to the duration of the Cancer Genetics Pilots Programme (three years).[2]

Who was in the NURG? Ironically, since some of the services were not yet fully up and running at the time of the events described, few of the 'users' had had a chance to use them. However, most of them were potential users on account of having a family history of cancer. Having such a history, as we discovered, took many forms. Some had lost loved ones to the disease, yet they had had to work hard to get information, screening or counselling. Others (those who had one of a number of specific genes, e.g. for breast or bowel cancer) knew they had an extremely high risk of getting cancer themselves. During an informal conversation before one of the NURG meetings we were struck by the story of one woman with a breast cancer gene who had chosen to have both her breasts removed to prevent her from developing breast cancer. All in all, these were people for whom this work mattered.

### A well-supported group

The NURG had a dedicated facilitator, funded by Macmillan. As well as convening the group's quarterly meetings in London, she supported members between meetings by speaking to them on the phone, ensuring their expenses were paid, and generally being there to listen and help out. The group also had an effective 'organisational sponsor' in the form of Macmillan senior manager Glyn Purland. He had been instrumental in negotiating with the Department of Health to get the Cancer Genetics Pilots Programme off the ground, and he held the Macmillan budget for the work throughout, participating in all the NURG meetings. Thus he acted as a permanent 'bridge' into the funding organisation. As we stress throughout this book, such a supporting team plays a vital part in sustaining the work of such a group. In this case, the team helped group members to contribute to the wider programme of work designed to benefit people with a family history of cancer. A narrative writer (Alison Donaldson) was also involved throughout the group's life, to track its progress and influence, and the meeting agendas always included a slot called 'narrative writing', in which there would be draft material to discuss. The conversations in this part of the meetings had a particular, free-flowing, storytelling quality about them and typically prompted members to go more deeply into their experiences. The more intimate quality of the talk stood out particularly from the more impersonal, transactional feeling of some of the other parts of the meetings.

### 'We have all had other lives'

One striking impression was the wide range of experience that members brought into the group. They included: a qualified librarian, an engineer-turned-web-designer, a former senior care assistant at a residential home, a software expert, a former civil servant, a former childcare lecturer, and someone who had taught all her adult life. As the ex-teacher put it:

> *Because we all have had other lives, and we all do have other skills, whatever they may be, we bring all of those to this new situation. I sometimes wonder whether some of the hesitancy of using patients and carers is because they don't actually know who these people are . . . they don't know where to pitch what they're talking about. So, I think it may be one of the things that we could contribute to a partnership. Instead of us remaining very anonymous – you know, 'I'm just a patient', or 'I'm just a carer', we ought to give them some indication of who we are. (group member)*

It also became clear how important it was for those members who had a professional background themselves (e.g. teacher, civil servant) not to get too drawn into treating the group as an extension of their own professional career but to stand in the shoes of potential service users. As another member put it:

> *You have to hold on to your own story and why you're there, which sometimes means stepping back a bit. I have found it's a constant battle not to jump in and be like*

*a professional because I have been one myself. You have to maintain your role as someone who has experienced this journey and remember there are other people who can do the professional bit. You have to value your own experience. (group member)*

In the quarterly meetings of the NURG, members shared a wide range of experiences and took what they learned back into their local area. In this way, ideas and insights from the group's conversations 'rippled out' via the people they spoke to after the meetings.

**Shaping priorities of pilot services**

At the beginning of its work as a group, the NURG was asked to review a comprehensive model (a document) that had been developed both to assess people's risk of getting cancer and to improve counselling services. In particular, they were asked to identify the model's 10 most important features from a service-user's perspective. The priorities identified were fed into the evaluations of the pilot projects and influenced the final reports. Members themselves stressed the value of this piece of work. One said that the group 'really gelled when we were given a task to do'.

**Patients involved as 'part of the team'**

One of the seven pilot sites (in Oldham) stood out as an example of what partnership working between service users and health professionals can look like when the circumstances are right. The two patients from Oldham (Carol and Jacqui) who came to the national group meetings had been attracted to the pilot project by their specialist breast nurse and genetics counsellor, Melanie Ripley, and they effectively became part of the team. For example, they helped present the project at events by literally standing alongside Melanie and telling their personal stories, explaining how they got involved with the cancer genetics service. They also helped the service make contact with 'hard-to-reach' communities, by running a stall during National Women's Week to promote the cancer genetics service among the local Asian community. And they even did fundraising for the service, which they wanted to see continuing to involve service users after the pilot phase, by raising funds and paying them into a specially created trust fund for this purpose. Melanie commented:

*They both brought their own unique talents and different lifetime experiences enriching both the service and the team. (Melanie Ripley)*

**Improving written information given to patients**

One way in which lay groups can be extremely helpful is in reviewing (or creating) literature designed to provide patients and carers with useful information. The value of this contribution quickly became apparent during the NURG meetings. For example, a university researcher came along to share some draft writing with the group, including an information sheet and interview guides for a study involving ethnic minority populations in Yorkshire. The researcher received a number of constructive suggestions about the text, and she remarked that she hadn't realised the extent to which she had been using technical language. On another occasion, a group member brought along a letter that GPs had sent out to some 100 people who had reported having cancer in their family. The draft letter included the sentence 'Our records indicate that you have a family history of cancer' and the group was quick to point out that this might alarm people unnecessarily. The project team subsequently amended the letter to reflect the group's comments. And someone from another charity (Cancerbackup, merged with Macmillan in 2008) who took part in many of the group's meetings commented:

> *Being part of the group helped me in my role of developing Cancerbackup's genetic information. One member was particularly helpful with my writing of information on risk-reducing breast surgery. But, in general, just hearing stories of personal experiences from all members of the group helped me to understand better the priorities and information needs of people using cancer genetic services. (group participant)*

Members commented that clinicians often thought they were being clear, but having a lay person involved helped health professionals develop more appropriate language. One person added that the issue was not just about clarity – in a leaflet, for example, certain phrases could easily upset people in a vulnerable situation.

### Attracting people from hard-to-reach population groups

Conversations in the national group also confirmed how difficult it can be to reach certain population groups, such as ethnic minorities and poor families. One particular incident involving people from the Leeds pilot project illustrates some of the challenges related to finding and supporting service-user representatives from such groups (*see* box).

#### Travelling across England to a group meeting in London

One of the explicit aims of the Leeds pilot project was to increase equity of access to cancer genetics services, particularly for people from ethnic minorities and poorer families. Initially it proved difficult finding patient advocates from these groups. But some months into the Cancer Genetics Pilots Programme, Liz Rowett (staff member and user involvement lead in the project) decided to use the contacts she had within her local Trust and to make a real effort to find individuals from ethnic minorities to join the project. She was put in contact with two women of Pakistani origin, one of whom knew her from her previous post as Clinical Nurse Specialist. Both agreed that they would be willing to join, though they seemed hesitant about travelling independently to London for the NURG meetings. Nevertheless, they agreed that they would be happy to go together by train.

When the date of the next NURG meeting in London arrived, Liz accompanied the two women all the way from Wakefield to Kings Cross and across London to the meeting at Macmillan's UK offices near Vauxhall. At the end of the day, she met up with them again for the journey home. (She particularly remembered them saying 'You won't leave us, will you?') The whole day involved extra travel for Liz, which she didn't mind because she felt a responsibility to people who had given up their time to take part in the project, and she wanted to make it as easy as possible for them to do so. And since she felt uncomfortable asking the two new representatives to buy their own tickets, Liz volunteered to purchase these herself and claim the money back from Macmillan:

*It is easy to say that we would like to recruit people from specific community or patient groups but this is not always straightforward. One of the issues that I feel needs to be brought to the fore is the financial one. . . . The train fare from Leeds to London with a one-day tube pass is just over £170. People usually purchase their own rail tickets and claim the money back from Macmillan. But I am not sure that people have £170 kicking around as spare cash to use on a train fare, and not everybody has a credit card and not everyone has the confidence that they would be reimbursed this money. I do think that organisations need to very carefully consider what type of support is required to encourage people to be comfortable in becoming patient representatives. (Liz Rowett, user involvement lead, Leeds pilot project)*

Other people have confirmed to us that health professionals often feel hesitant or uncomfortable about asking patients to get involved in groups or projects to help the NHS improve its services. They may fear that they will be placing a burden on people who already have health and sometimes also psychological problems. Patients may say 'yes' in order to please the nurse who has looked after them. Moreover, health professionals may feel particularly protective towards patients who live within a different ethnic community and may therefore be less well travelled, may need to get permission from family members or elders, and may not be used to talking openly about cancer, let alone the possibility of their own family having a history of the disease. And finally, the patients whose voice is most needed may be those who have no contact whatsoever with the health professional in question.

### Responding to difficult group dynamics

Reflecting on the experience of being in the NURG, members said that it had become a source of great support and had boosted their self-confidence, but there was one exception, and that person stopped attending the meetings within the first months. This was a reminder that joining a group can be a daunting experience and that comments intended constructively can sometimes be heard as criticism. In general, however, the NURG meetings felt warm and supportive, once the membership stabilised (which happened within a few meetings). A community facilitator with the right skills and experience can respond to such complex group dynamics and help maintain the group spirit.

## PORTRAIT: SARAH'S PERSONAL AND PROFESSIONAL CONTRIBUTION

The person who came to the NURG quarterly meetings from the Teesside pilot project was a retired school teacher, who asked us to refer to her as Sarah. Sarah contributed both personal experience and professional expertise to the programme. Before we met her, she had cared for four people and had also been a volunteer with Samaritans (a UK charity that provides emotional support for people who are experiencing feelings of distress or despair). Professionally, she had taught all her life and had recently been running workshops for teachers in continental Europe.

Asked to reflect on what motivates people to get involved in a group, she said:

> *Fear comes into it quite a lot, whether it is the experience of having had cancer or of being the one who has to manage the situation and make huge decisions as a carer. When people come out the other side of such an experience, they want to use their new knowledge to help other people. They want to clarify things and make it easier for others who may be going through uncertainty and confusion.* (Sarah)

Sarah had the advantage of being involved with the Teesside pilot project from its inception. As a member of the local partnership group, she helped with the bid for pilot service funding. And once the proposal was accepted, she helped draw up criteria for appointing professionals to run the service and was present at the interviews. Soon after this, Sarah and other people living with cancer took part with professionals in a workshop about how the service should be run. The pilot lead (a hospital consultant) commented afterwards that he 'never thought he would get so much from a user group'.

Even though Sarah's mother, aunt and sister had all died of cancer, when she became involved in the Cancer Genetics Pilots Programme she hadn't yet used the genetics service, so she decided to refer herself. So the service was investigating Sarah's family medical records while we were working on this portrait. This prompted her to make a constructive suggestion about the assessment process: when people are assessed, they are placed in categories, one of which is 'low risk';

but given that one in three members of the population gets cancer during their lifetime, Sarah suggested that it might be more accurate to use the term 'low genetic risk' for this particular category.

Sarah's previous experience of teaching and running workshops proved particularly useful to her local cancer genetics service. In December 2005, the pilot service had seen nearly 2000 patients, so the moment was opportune to do some evaluation. However, the project team were nervous of the extra work that face-to-face interviews would create, so Sarah suggested they could instead run a workshop, with refreshments provided and professionals present. At this event, patients would be asked to share their thoughts and could also be invited to help form a patient group. This would enable the project team to demonstrate that service-user involvement had made a positive contribution to the pilot service and had not just been a token effort.

The project team also benefited from hearing what Sarah and her fellow patients and carers had to say about questionnaires and letters *before* these were sent to patients. Sarah suggested that these materials should be viewed not just singly but as a series of communications and that, after returning a filled-in questionnaire, people should always get a 'thank you' and some indication of how long it will be before they hear again and why it may take a while. Otherwise, people often experience several months silence, not realising the time it takes to investigate a family history.

We can see from Sarah's story that, just because people take part in a community of influence as 'lay members', this does not mean they have no professional expertise to contribute. Sarah's background in teaching, as well as her personal experience and self-confidence, enabled her to make many constructive suggestions to her local cancer genetics service. She was then able to share her knowledge and ideas by taking part in the NURG meetings.

Patients and carers clearly have to strike a balance between being there as someone who has gone through a particular experience with illness, and as someone with whatever skills and expertise they happen to have.

## HOW MUCH SUPPORT DO PATIENT GROUPS NEED?

During a period of restructuring and review, touched upon elsewhere in this book, Macmillan disbanded the group of people living with cancer that had been set up to inform its work with doctors, and started moving towards a different form of partnership working. By now the charity had access to an extensive network of Cancer Voices.[3] So, instead of continuing to invest in working with a small group of people living with cancer, as before, Macmillan started sending out an open invitation to the Cancer Voices to take part in the GP meetings.

Without a community facilitator, there was nobody who really knew how to prepare patients and carers to work in partnership with health professionals. The kind of situations that arose included people turning up who were still in active treatment, or who didn't know that 'death' was a topic likely to come up. Some of the GPs even ended up comforting some of the Cancer Voices who became upset during the conference. Fortunately, in 2008 Lorraine was brought back again to work with what was now an enlarged Macmillan Primary Care Community (for the story of how this evolved out of the Macmillan GP Community, *see* Chapter 3). With time, she was able to shed her other responsibilities and focus on this now sizeable community of influence. To help prepare the Cancer Voices taking part in community meetings, Lorraine developed formal selection criteria and an informative briefing letter. The 2010 Primary Care Conference was a better experience as a result, though some challenges remained, as we shall see shortly.

Thus, by 2010 an interesting juncture had been reached in the way Macmillan worked with its 'lay communities of influence'. The relationship between community members and the sponsoring organisation had become more distant. Also, there was little appetite within the organisation to return to funding what were seen as costly smaller groups of people living with cancer. Even Lorraine, as an experienced community facilitator, acknowledged that working in that way had sometimes meant she ended up spending a good deal of time 'managing relationships within the group'. In addition, Macmillan proposed to limit people's involvement to two years maximum, in order to be sure of bringing in 'fresh blood'.

### Two different models of user involvement

There are pros and cons to each approach – a small, well-supported group versus a wider network of Cancer Voices. As we have seen, the smaller groups, which bonded and met over a prolonged period, offered people a 'safe environment' in which they could exchange experiences and develop a collective voice. However, there were risks: people might become disillusioned and spread negative stories if their personal interests weren't given priority; or it might become too easy to predict what certain individuals were going to say.

The Cancer Voices model was more inclusive and less costly, but it came with its own risks. New people joining would not have the benefit of the safe environment of a small group, and when they joined the Primary Care Community a few apparently made anti-GP or otherwise inappropriate remarks. Macmillan's former User Involvement Advisor Jane Bradburn expressed the dilemma well:

> *Personally my view is that the development of a looser, wider Cancer Voices network was inevitable, as the original approach was very time consuming, expensive and just didn't involve enough people in terms of quantity and diversity. We ended*

*up with the same people on all the different committees and groups. However, an experienced, trained Cancer Voice, used to working with health professionals, makes the work more productive and the lay person feels more supported. (Jane Bradburn)*

### Value of mature relationships

Whichever approach prevails in future, to date many of the members of the Macmillan lay communities of influence remain actively linked to the charity. In a few cases a 'mature relationship' developed between a lay person, the funding organisation and the communities of health professionals. For example, in Chapter 5 we described how Roberta Lovick took part as a lay member in a group of clinician researchers ('hybrid creatures') over a number of years and was able to exercise a strong influence on the choice of research topics and their relevance to quality of care.

Some of the Cancer Voices continued to participate in Macmillan's Primary Care Conferences. Some also took part each year in the National Cancer Research Institute's conferences, where they helped create an annual competition for patient-led research. This competition became well established, and before long Macmillan was funding about three patient-led studies each year, with patients doing some of the field research. The whole idea continued to grow, so that by 2008 there were proposals actually written by patients.

## POINTS TO CONSIDER WHEN INVOLVING LAY PEOPLE

There is plenty of practical advice publicly available on how to set up and run self-help and partnership groups.[4] What we offer below are a few issues that matter when the main purpose of a lay community is to influence and improve services.

### The people

*People who live with cancer are experts by experience. (Macmillan Cancer Support website)*[5]

The patients and carers we have described had generally experienced some distressing event, such as the death of a loved one or a cancer diagnosis, and it was often this that propelled them into lending their experience and support to others facing similar problems. This provides a clue about how government, voluntary organisations and citizens might increasingly work together in future in ways that none of these parties could do as well alone.

There has been some debate about whether people who get involved in these kinds of activities are 'representative' of patients as a whole. We think that it is more helpful to think about *perspectives*.[6] Members of the public are invited to join a group mainly to provide a perspective that is distinctive from that of health professionals. They have either been patients themselves or have cared for a sick person.

Carers (family, friends or colleagues who look after a person living with a serious or chronic disability or illness like cancer) bring with them their own issues and are viewed by some as the 'unsung heroes' in healthcare. When people are actively caring, that is usually all they have time for, so they tend not to get involved in influencing-work until later. But the experience of caring for a dying person remains present for such people and informs their participation in a community of influence. As one carer said: 'Once you're a carer you're always a carer, because it's never ever going to leave you.'

### The 'group advantage'

The groups we have described in this chapter were typically made up of about 12–15 people who met regularly to pursue an overall aim proposed by the sponsoring organisation. Working as part of such a group, rather than ploughing a lone furrow, had a number of advantages. From the members' point of view, there was the benefit of company and support of other people who could empathise with their experience yet offer a different perspective.

In addition, we have heard members report that being part of a group gave them greater confidence, enabling them to 'speak out' in other settings. (For example, the former teacher, Sarah, mentioned earlier, said she had always been used to addressing children but suddenly found herself as the second speaker after a professor in a lecture theatre, and she felt very proud when she had got through it.) People also told us that, by being part of a group, they came to feel less like a 'token user' and more respected and listened to – they felt it gave them authority. And saying that they were part of a Macmillan group seemed to provoke interest among people they spoke to.

### Judging the moment to get involved in an influencing group.

Involving patients or carers in an influencing group clearly poses particular challenges, e.g. judging the amount of time that should have lapsed since diagnosis or bereavement before getting involved, and being mindful that patients in particular may be experiencing continuing illness and treatment.

There is no 'right time' for patients or carers to get involved – it depends so much on individual circumstances. One patient in the cancer genetics NURG was particularly pleased to have been in at the beginning so she could have an influence on the service as it developed. Another also found the timing was good for her, but for a different reason – a couple of years earlier and she would have been caught up in dealing with her own cancer diagnosis and treatment. In general, members agreed that anyone who had lost someone to cancer typically needed at least 12 months before participating in such a group.

### A collective aim but a flexible agenda

As we stress throughout this book, a community of influence is different from the average team or working group, and cannot be 'managed' in the same way. One of the group facilitators we worked with expressed it well:

> *You can have an overall aim, a big picture, but to put too much detail around that is going to hinder the project. If you are working with users, they put the flesh on the bone, and they may redirect the original aim that you had, and that doesn't matter. (community facilitator)*

When a group starts to meet, there may be formal terms of reference, but we have found that they tend to remain in the background. It is, above all, the conversations, stories, relationships and community facilitator that make the difference.

### Working on concrete tasks

We find that a 'joint inquiry' with a specific purpose helps give a group focus and can be very satisfying for members (this holds for both lay and professional groups). It also increases the chances of a tangible product coming into existence that can in turn be used to influence policy and practice.

A good example was the booklet created in 2004 by an 'expert carer group' set up by Macmillan to influence its work in social care.[7] *Hello and How Are You?* turned out to be a very popular Macmillan publication. People who had come out of a situation of despair and turned it into something positive, as one member put it, felt it was 'quite a privilege' to create something that could help others in a similar situation. One carer spoke particularly movingly about the satisfaction she had gained from working on the booklet:

> *One of the promises my husband extracted from me in the last weeks of his life was he made me promise I wouldn't sit around on my backside wallowing in self-pity, I would get out into the community and do something positive. He didn't say what that positive thing had got to be, but I feel this has given me the opportunity to fulfil his wish. And that means more to me than anything. (person living with cancer)*

### Preparing lay people for partnership with health professionals

As we have seen, people living with cancer were invited to take part in the meetings of the Macmillan-sponsored communities of influence made up mainly of health professionals, to keep the discussions grounded in the needs and priorities of patients. To make this kind of partnership a success, thorough preparation proved vital. In our experience, this is best done by a community facilitator who understands how communities of influence work, has sensible criteria for judging whether someone is ready to take part in meetings with health professionals, and knows how to brief and support them. Several people commented particularly on the Macmillan-funded courses for Cancer Voices, which, they said, help people learn that user involvement is about developing a group voice to improve things for people living with cancer, not about 'trying to change everything because of your personal experience of being diagnosed with cancer'.

### Handling 'exits' with care

Lay groups can be difficult to keep together. Illness or carer responsibilities may prevent people from participating continuously. Or some may find it hard to understand the difference between contributing a lay perspective (which is what they are there to do) and 'representing' patients (which is *not* their role). Another potential problem is that certain members may bring up the same hobby horse time and again. For all these reasons it is important to find ways of recognising when the time has come for someone to move on.

One way of enabling people to leave a group feeling acknowledged and satisfied is to invite them to spend a bit of time acting as mentor and support for new people joining (as mentioned in Chapter 7). In addition, the community facilitator can play an important part in showing that the individual's contribution has been appreciated. It is also worth considering whether membership should be time limited (perhaps two or three years), so that fresh perspectives can be regularly brought into the group. A few members may become tired or disillusioned and the worst thing that can happen is that they leave the group feeling bitter and then spread negative gossip about it.

### How much support?

In Chapter 6 we explored more fully the kinds of support that can help to make communities of influence productive and sustainable. We can see from the Macmillan examples that a considerable investment was made in its lay communities – as well as facilitation and support, members were usually offered training and reimbursement of expenses. Some key questions remain for organisations wanting to sponsor this kind of partnership working; for example, is there enough funding to invest in a dedicated group of lay people? This may seem costly to maintain, but it can act as a community of influence in its own right and also bring a patient voice into the meetings of the communities made up mainly of health professionals.

Whether the decision is to go for a small, intensively supported group or a looser network, some degree of support (e.g. a community facilitator) will help make sure that patients and carers are well prepared for their engagement with professional communities of influence.[8]

## NOTES

1 Macmillan's work with doctors was known as its 'medical strategy', but the charity also had a 'user involvement strategy'. So the creation of lay groups to inform its work with doctors was in effect linked to both strands of work. In 2001, Jane Bradburn, who featured in Chapter 1, joined Macmillan as User Involvement Advisor and helped to develop a user involvement strategy. It had three main strands: (i) helping the NHS set up Partnership Groups in 31 of 34 new cancer networks in England; (ii) further developing the UK-wide Cancer Voices network (people living with cancer who were prepared to work as volunteers), which she had helped create in her previous job; and (iii) establishing lay involvement in all key areas of activity within Macmillan, including research, social care, information, education and the medical strategy.

2 Donaldson A, Lank E, Maher J. Sharing experiences of user involvement in shaping new services: the story of a national patient group. *Familial Cancer*. 2007; **6**(2): 249–56.

3 www.macmillan.org.uk/GetInvolved/CancerVoices/CancerVoices.aspx (23 December 2010).

4 www.macmillan.org.uk/HowWeCanHelp/CancerSupportGroups/CancerSupportGroups.aspx (23 December 2010).

5 www.macmillan.org.uk/Aboutus/WhatWeDo/What_we_do.aspx (23 December 2010).

6 Bradburn J, Maher J. Editorial: user and carer participation in research in palliative care. *Palliative Medicine*. 2005; **19**(2): 91–2.

7 www.macmillan.org.uk/Documents/Hello%20and%20how%20are%20you.pdf (23 December 2010).

8 One option considered earlier but rejected by Macmillan was for patient and carer advocates to be an independent body, separate from the organisation and its professional communities of influence. This is evidently the practice in some countries and it obviously spares the organisation the cost of supporting lay people, but it brings with it other disadvantages.

CHAPTER 8

# Playing a long game

## Benefits and risks of working with communities of influence over time

### OVERVIEW

*Working with communities of influence is not a one-off initiative. It involves identifying credible and influential individuals, keeping groups and relationships alive over time, recognising that individuals will come and go, and being prepared to rekindle relationships when the circumstances are right, or otherwise part ways satisfactorily. All of this takes time and requires negotiation and patience rather than control and short-term thinking. Hence the phrase 'playing a long game'.*

*As we reflected on our experience, what crystallised for us was that working with communities of influence means, first and foremost, taking relationships and conversations seriously. It also requires rethinking a whole range of assumptions, related for example, to how we think about outcomes, and what kind of skills and resources are needed. Anyone setting out on this journey will need to articulate the value of this way of working to cost-conscious managers. But if people and organisations do develop the capacity to work with communities of influence and nurture long-term relationships, we believe they will be developing a vital and valuable capability that can help improve policy and practice over the long term.*

While working on this book, we dedicated some time to reflecting together on what further insights have emerged for us and which themes we think need highlighting in the complex work of cultivating communities of influence.

## LONG-TERM RELATIONSHIPS AT THE CENTRE OF THE WORK

The central theme of the work, all three of us quickly agreed, remained a focus on long-term relationships, i.e. connections and conversations. For the more business-minded among our readers, the phrase 'relationships as an asset' may hit the mark. In other words, relationships are worth paying attention to, valuing and maintaining like any other form of 'capital'.

Working in this way means taking a long-term view. So, during the early months of a community's life, when tangible results may be hard to identify, everybody involved may need extra patience and perseverance. Part of the role of the supporting team in the early days, therefore, is to encourage people to understand that it will take time to get to know one another and develop a common sense of purpose, and that this is just as important as the more tangible products and results achieved in the community's first year:

> *I have been working with a new community for the past few months and I have been struck by the tension within the group between the need to give time to getting to know one another and the urge to agree some kind of common purpose as quickly as possible.* (Alison)

One of the most important elements of the initial months is developing trust or 'bonding'. This is not just an agreeable experience. It also makes productive collaboration much easier. Community members become more likely to think of one another when, for example, they are looking for someone to talk through a clinical issue, join them in a project, share a keynote speech, or partner them in a visit to a senior policymaker. As one community member commented: 'Because you develop relationships, you can ask each other favours more easily.'

A word of caution: while trust and goodwill take time to develop, they can be lost rapidly if the sponsoring organisation is inattentive or unsupportive. The good news, though, is that, provided there is no major rupture or falling out, the relationships and trust that grow up between people can live on for years and often outlast both the official existence of the community and the hierarchical structures of the organisations it is there to influence.

## TAKING CONVERSATION SERIOUSLY

We revealed our own interest in conversation and storytelling in Chapter 2, but we do recognise that not everybody shares our views on this. Indeed, when initially invited to participate in communities of influence, people sometimes say: 'I'm concerned this will just be a talking shop'.

However, it is worth repeating that anybody who really pays attention to conversation – that most everyday form of human interaction – is likely to start noticing how it can generate learning, novelty and influence. It can give rise to unpredictable insights and outcomes. As people exchange experiences and thoughts, new ideas can emerge as if 'out of the blue'. They may go away from a conversation feeling 'reorientated'. Yet the ubiquity and familiarity of conversation mean that we tend to take it for granted. It is so much under our noses that we seldom think about it. Furthermore, the 'results' of a conversation may not be immediately obvious – insights often take time to become clear.

> *We talk, we utter words, and only later do we get a picture of their life. (Ludwig Wittgenstein)*[1]

We have noticed for example that, if we are attentive to our thoughts for a few days after a community meeting, we often realise that something has shifted in our thinking, or that we are reusing a phrase that we first heard in the meeting. Phrases that linger in our minds can be thought of as 'vivid reminders'. These obviously differ for each group, but with time they can become part of the 'common language' that emerges between people. Indeed, in talking and writing about communities of influence, we have found ourselves adopting certain key phrases, such as 'making the invisible visible' and 'the social life of documents'. These expressions only emerged as we started working together, but we quickly noticed that people picked them up and started using them in their own ways and their own contexts.

We also recognise the part that emotions (e.g. anxiety, rivalry) and power differences play in conversation. These aspects of human relating have major consequences, especially for the team supporting a community of influence. For example, community members may feel anxious or impatient about the time it takes to agree a common purpose, or they may suspect that the funding organisation has a 'hidden agenda'. They do not always express these feelings directly. Whether members do or do not give voice to their concerns, those facilitating community meetings will do well to respond to them in some way. For example, sometimes it pays off to ease people's anxiety, e.g. by including some time for 'traditional' meeting activities (e.g. a discussion of a member's project, or a visit from an expert from outside the group). This may encourage community members to be more receptive to spending other parts of the meeting in a more reflective conversation. At other times it may be important to challenge people. Dealing with these complex aspects of human communication and influence requires empathy, judgement and nerve on the part of both community members and those supporting them.

If we think conversations and what emerges from them are important, it makes sense to pay attention to their *quality*. But what makes for a good conversation? It would of course take pages and pages to answer this question properly, but one factor that often seems to go unnoticed or unacknowledged is that of skilful 'convening'. All too often people follow the stale formula of packed agendas, one-way presentations and minimal time for productive conversation between people. In contrast, when meetings are designed as 'collaborative inquiries', encouraging people to share experiences and build relationships, the results can be both satisfying and productive. However, it does require considerable skill in convening, which includes paying attention to both meeting design and what emerges during the meeting, bearing in mind that with communities of influence, the locus of control needs to shift somewhat – from those who call the meeting to the other participants.

## RETHINKING THE NATURE OF 'OUTCOMES' AND 'OUTPUTS'

As mentioned elsewhere in this book, over time we came to articulate more precisely the kind of outcomes we saw emerging from communities of influence – in one sense, much of the output of conversations is simply 'more conversations'. People go off after a meeting and talk to their contacts, who in turn talk to their contacts, and so on, until the number reached is much larger than just the people in the original conversation. We began to refer to the stories, insights and ideas that spread and get amplified through successive conversations as 'ripple effects':

> *The participants in the original conversation may have no idea who is subsequently inspired by ideas that may have travelled through a lengthy chain of human exchanges. They never see the most distant ripple. (Alison)*

As we have seen, we also found ourselves coining the phrase 'knowledge products' to describe the tangible products or documents created by communities of influence. The measure of success for these products is not the creation of the document but the influence it has – which is all too often not tracked over time. Indeed, by talking about knowledge as a product, one risks falling into the common trap of reifying or, to use another term, 'thingifying' flow and movement. In knowledge management circles, people have tried to emphasise movement by talking about 'mobilising knowledge', but even that expression implies that knowledge is a thing. One useful discipline, we have found, is to seek to replace nouns with verbs or whole phrases wherever possible, e.g. talk about 'influencing' or 'sharing experiences', rather than 'influence' or 'knowledge'.

The message about community 'outcomes' that we want to leave with readers is that the difficulty of measuring them in precise, quantifiable terms should not be used as a reason for not investing in this way of working. Rather, we urge people to take up the challenge of creating meaningful, qualitative evaluation methods that take complexity into account. This includes thinking hard about the nature of 'outcomes'.

## HARDER TO DO THAN SOME MIGHT THINK

In talking to people about this work, we came across some who thought they were already doing what we were painstakingly trying to describe. This may be because things like conversation, relationships and communities seem so familiar to people, or it may be because people are just steeped in taken-for-granted ways of managing groups, meetings and projects. Below we highlight some of the challenges we encountered, starting with how to select suitable people to join a new group.

### Identifying suitable members for a community

> *Many people talk about building relationships but they don't really know how to do it. For example, the normal way of thinking about forming a group revolves around 'equity not cherry picking'. Yet our experience has been that 'cherry picking' can be very helpful. When we tried to form a community more 'democratically', it didn't work as well. (Jane)*

Clearly, when seeking new members for a community, what is needed is individuals with energy and commitment. This is something we can all recognise in people. The danger of a purist democratic selection process is that people may suggest members not on the basis of their energy and drive, but because they are seen to 'represent' a certain group, point of view or position in the organisational hierarchy.

### Challenges of working with strong characters

Another aspect of cultivating communities that may seem counter-intuitive to some is the value of having one or more strong personalities in a group:

> *Some people are frightened of bringing in mavericks. What they fail to realise is that the group helps to bring these people down to earth. If such a person can convince the group, there is a good chance they will be able to convince others. (Jane)*

In other words, the group can act as a testing ground for ideas and develop a kind of 'collective wisdom'. A broad diversity of experience and perspective in the group increases the chances that useful ideas will emerge from it. However it does often call on the skill of the supporting team to keep relationships and group discussions constructive and productive, when influential or charismatic individuals are putting forward strong views.

### Encouraging busy professionals to give time to reflection

Community meetings provide people with a space where they can explore their experience with others and discover new possibilities for their work as practitioners and influencers. However, often the kind of professionals who join communities of influence are extremely busy individuals not used to taking time out to reflect on their work and their lives. So we generally found that we needed to help people to reflect on their experience, e.g. by setting aside time for them to explore 'How well are we working together?' – and the best time to do this was during community meetings:

> *I think people lack 'brain space' outside the meetings. We wanted them to continue talking and emailing between meetings, but they sometimes felt overwhelmed. (Jane)*

Given the importance of the community meetings as a 'space for reflection', the person brought in to make the conversations productive (the convenor) became very important in enabling groups to strike a balance between discussing 'content' and reflecting on 'process'.

### In-house vs. external skills

In the communities described in this book, there was always a supporting team, including roles like community sponsor, community facilitator, clinical lead and external consultants. As external consultants, Alison and Elizabeth were responsible (among other things) for designing productive meetings and tracking the group's life using narrative writing. Talking about the skills assembled in the supporting group, Jane commented:

> *We all agreed that some roles are better in-house – for example, the community sponsor and facilitator roles. Those people need to know the organisation inside out, which means being familiar with the people, the politics, the strategic aims, the way things are done, and so on. Some of the other community development roles involve skills that are not normally found in-house, or if they are, it can be more cost-effective to bring external people in when needed. For example, the work needs a special kind of writer who not only has the narrative writing skills but understands and is interested in this kind of work. And designing and facilitating effective community meetings often requires some external expertise. These are big investments but don't require full-time support. (Jane)*

### Knowing the risks involved and how to deal with them

Despite the value of community conversations, there are also considerable risks, worth knowing about and even anticipating if possible. A common one is trying to over-manage a community.

Other key risks relate to the lifecycle of the community. The examples in this book have been mainly about how we created and sustained communities of influence, but it is also worth thinking about when the time might have arrived to wind down such an investment.

Community members tend to go through intense experiences together, develop strong relationships and grow more confident as influencers. One risk is that, having empowered people in this way, the funding organisation may 'drop them' when the initial funding period ends or organisational sponsors move on. Since group members are not employees of the funding organisation, the challenge is to maintain some kind of connection if funding is interrupted or discontinued, or at least find ways of tracking relationships that continue naturally elsewhere.

Another risk is that those community members who develop into national leaders begin to find they can 'go direct to the top' by speaking to policymakers. In doing so, they may not acknowledge the support of the organisation that invested in their influencing role in the first place. Indeed, they may no longer feel they need the community, except as an instrument or a source of information. The funding organisation can either seek to make continued involvement in the community satisfying for these highly influential members, which might mean giving them more of a leadership role within the community, or it can work to keep an ongoing relationship with them outside the community. In any case, community membership will inevitably change over time and as influential contributors move on to other things, new members with fresh ideas can be invited in to take their place.

## ARTICULATING THIS WAY OF WORKING TO HARD-NOSED MANAGERS

> *One thing that I think is really important, and there isn't any other way to do it, is changing the way people view things by changing the way they talk about them, and that's something I've observed these groups doing over time. New ways of looking at things emerge and get amplified. This changes the conversation and can then be used to prepare the ground for useful products. (Jane)*

We end this book in a sense where it began: with the need to continue helping those who hold the purse strings to 'get it' – to understand how communities of influence work and what they contribute. Of the three authors of this book, Jane (as a senior member of the funding organisation) was always under the most pressure to demonstrate the 'so what?' – the value of investing in communities of influence, of nurturing long-term relationships and taking conversations and connections seriously. She never ceased 'scratching away at' this by asking 'will a hard-nosed commissioning person or budget holder accept the outcomes we are pointing to?'

### Combining numbers, concepts, stories and pictures

Given the need to continue articulating how communities of influence work and what they contribute, we are always thinking hard about which forms of communication work best in which situations and with which people. In our experience, this means using every form of communication. With time, we found that, depending on the person we were trying to influence, a *combination* of concepts, stories, numbers and pictures was helpful in explaining what we were trying to do and helping people to 'get it'. For example, at certain points in time, pictures became important in enabling policymakers to grasp a new or different way of doing things; at other times those responsible for funding needed to see figures, such as the number of publications produced by our hybrid research group (*see* Chapter 5).

From time to time we discussed whether videos or pictures were more persuasive than writing, but we remain convinced that writing has an important place in describing and recording the work of communities. The great advantage of 'writing it down' is that people can always go back to the written word and use it to stimulate further thinking, dialogue and, in some cases, to inspire action. Writing also provides a document that endures and can be 'pointed to' as tangible evidence of results.

### Using funding wisely

In Chapter 6 we showed what kind and level of resources may be needed to sustain a community of influence. Jane reflected on what she felt she had learned about how to time and structure the funding to attract excellent people and keep them engaged in the community:

> *The money is important in that it helps to attract good people. But I am beginning to think that perhaps we should fund communities in phases. The first would be about developing the community – the money would pay for backfill for the health professionals, travel and accommodation, plus the external consultants needed to help build the community and do the narrative tracking. The second phase would focus more on projects and project funding, with less money being needed for supporting the group. And there might be a third phase, after the projects are completed, when tracking and facilitation become more important again.* (Jane)

### Is this really a 'new' approach?

When testing and articulating a particular way of working, it is easy to fall into the trap of describing it as 'new'. The risk of claiming to have a new way is that it can turn people off. Also, they naturally tend to relate what you are saying to something they know already. In many ways, the community activities we have been writing about – conversation, storytelling, sharing experiences and spreading ideas – seem familiar and unremarkable to most people. They are normal activities in any community of human beings.

> *I am wondering if it's actually an old approach rather than a new one – human societies have been operating this way for ever, but ordinary human behaviour has become subverted by managerial and rational thinking. Perhaps what we are doing is simply tapping into 'how people are' to make things happen. (Elizabeth)*

We are also aware that many other people (e.g. in the fields of organisational development and executive coaching) have been highlighting the importance of relationships, dialogue and community for years, albeit using slightly different language from ours.

Academics have also written about such topics. For example, the concept of a 'resourceful community', introduced by Shotter and Katz,[2] is very close to our term 'communities of influence'. In both cases, community members share striking moments and memorable experiences, develop new ways of talking, discover what knowledge and expertise they can draw on from the group, and form lasting relationships that enable them to accomplish more together. In other words, they do much more than exchange information – they make connections and create a resourceful community or pool of knowledge upon which they can draw in their influencing roles.

## COMMUNITY BUILDING: A VITAL ORGANISATIONAL CAPABILITY

Whether readers judge the ways of working we have been describing as new or old, we suggest that the best organisations in future will recognise the power of the collective voice and the value of long-term relationships. Certainly in the health sector there is much talk about how to provide patients with joined-up care. Working with communities of influence, *without* having direct authority over community members, could help to make this a reality. We hope the ideas and experiences we have shared here will encourage and stimulate others who choose to embark on a similar journey. We think they will be developing one of the vital organisational capabilities of the future.

## NOTES

1 Wittgenstein L. *Philosophical Investigations.* 1953; p. 209. Cited in: Shotter J, Katz AM. Articulating a practice from within the practice itself: establishing formative dialogues by the use of a 'social poetics'. *Concepts and Transformation.* 1996; **1**(2/3): 213–37.

2 Katz AM, Siegel BS, Rappo P. Reflections from a collaborative pediatric mentorship program: building a community of resources. *Ambulatory Child Health.* 1997; **3**: 101–12. See also: Katz AM, Shotter J. Resonances from within the practice: social poetics in a mentorship program. *Concepts and Transformation.* 1996; **2**: 97–105.

POSTSCRIPT

# A writer's personal reflections

**Alison Donaldson**

*We record stories of what we are doing and what others around us are doing and as we develop these, the themes of the research emerge. This is why it is only clear what we have been doing when we are almost finished doing it. (Ralph Stacey, email communication)*

As one of the authors about to finish working on this book, I find it impossible to resist the temptation to use writing – again – to reflect on what it has all meant and where it might lead next. I often think back to where this journey began. Of course, it is impossible to isolate one beginning for any complex set of experiences, but one of the beginnings for us was back in 2003 when I mentioned to Jane Maher that the main method of my just-completed doctoral research had been 'reflective narrative writing'. I recall at the time thinking this would sound very academic and specialised, so I was surprised when Jane said 'That sounds interesting'. Little did I know that that was the beginning of a long collaborative working relationship with both Jane and Elizabeth, which would lead to this book.

In relation to the narrative writing, some particularly arresting moments have stayed with me. One was when, on hearing about the group of patients and carers that had introduced the document they had created (*Our Principles of People-Centred Care*) to dozens of people, I suddenly saw a connection with my own doctoral research and found myself enthusiastically proposing to write an account called 'The social life of a document'. Chapter 4 of this book grew out of this key moment.

Another was the spontaneous and excited response of the editor of the *Journal of Change Management* when he received our draft article called 'Making the invisible visible' – this was our first attempt at expressing our thinking on the challenge of evaluating complex human endeavours, which has now found its way into Chapter 2.

A third occurred at a meeting with another group of patients and carers. It was 7 July 2005, the day of the 7/7 London bombings, and only three of us had made it to the meeting, which would normally have involved about 15. Phone calls quickly revealed that the others were not going to make it – most had been forced to turn round and go home. So there we were, wondering whether to stay and talk to each other or try to get home, probably with difficulty. We decided to stay until lunchtime, eat some of the sandwiches meant for 15 people and give the rest away to staff who happened to be in the building. This was when I got into conversation with the woman who had chosen to have both her breasts removed because the breast cancer gene in her family meant that she was extremely likely, if not certain, to get cancer otherwise. It gave me a shocking glimpse of the kind of life experiences that lay behind some people's participation in these groups.

As the book writing draws to a close, I have less a sense of ending and more of beginning again. We are ready now to talk to a wider circle of people about the work, and especially to engage with those who are interested in what voluntary organisations, practitioners and ordinary citizens can all do to make a difference in their chosen field. I hope that the stories we have told and the arguments we have put forward in this book will be stimulating and useful to those we want to reach – busy but reflective managers and practitioners. I would like to leave readers with an apt quote from Jerome Bruner:

> *A good story and a well-formed argument are different natural kinds. Both can be used as means for convincing another. Yet what they convince of is fundamentally different: arguments convince one of their truth, stories of their lifelikeness. (Jerome Bruner)*[1]

## NOTE

1 Bruner J. *Actual Minds, Possible Worlds.* Cambridge, MA and London: Harvard University Press; 1986. pp. 11–43.

# Suggestions for further reading

## ON COMMUNITIES AND NETWORKS

- Collison C, Parcell G. *Learning to Fly: practical knowledge management from leading and learning organizations*. Chichester: Capstone/Wiley; 2004.
- Cross R, Parker A. *The Hidden Power of Social Networks: understanding how work really gets done in organizations*. Boston: Harvard Business School Publishing; 2004.
- Lank E. *Collaborative Advantage: how organizations win by working together*. Basingstoke: Palgrave Macmillan; 2006.
- Wenger E. *Communities of Practice: learning, meaning and identity*. Cambridge: Cambridge University Press; 1998.
- Wenger E, McDermott R, Snyder W. *Cultivating Communities of Practice: a guide to managing knowledge*. Boston, MA: Harvard Business School Press; 2002.

## ON COMPLEXITY AND EMERGENCE

- Shaw P. *Changing Conversations in Organizations: a complexity approach to change*. London and New York: Routledge; 2002.
- Stacey R. *Experiencing Emergence in Organizations: local interaction and the emergence of global pattern*. London: Routledge; 2005.
- Stacey R. *Strategic Management and Organisational Dynamics: the challenge of complexity*. 5th ed. Harlow, Essex: Prentice Hall; 2007.
- Waldrop MM. *Complexity: the emerging science at the edge of order and chaos*. London: Penguin Books; 1992.

## ON WRITING AND NARRATIVE

- Bruner J. *Actual Minds, Possible Worlds*. Cambridge, MA and London: Harvard University Press; 1986. pp. 11–43.
- Carr EH. *What is History?* London: Penguin Books; 1990 (first published 1961).
- Clandinin DJ, Connelly FM. *Narrative Inquiry: experience and story in qualitative research*. San Francisco: Jossey-Bass; 2000.

- Clifford J, Marcus GE. *Writing Culture: the poetics and politics of ethnography.* Berkeley and Los Angeles, CA: University of California Press; 1986.
- Czarniawska B. *A Narrative Approach to Organization Studies.* London: SAGE Publications; 1998.
- Donaldson A. *Reflexive writing and the social life of documents.* Paper presented at the 23rd Colloquium of the European Group for Organizational Studies, Vienna University, July 2007. Available from alison@writinginorganisations.co.uk
- Evans RJ. *In Defence of History.* London: Granta Publications; 1997.
- Geertz C. *Works and Lives: the anthropologist as author.* Cambridge: Polity Press; 1988.
- Gergen KJ. *An Invitation to Social Constructionism.* London: SAGE Publications; 1999 (reprinted 2000).
- Lakoff G, Johnson M. *Metaphors We Live By.* Chicago: University of Chicago Press; 1980.
- Polkinghorne DE. *Narrative Knowing and the Human Sciences.* New York: State University of New York Press; 1988.
- Rhodes C, Brown AD. Narrative, organizations and research. *International Journal of Management Reviews.* 2005; 7(3): 167–88.
- Scholes RE, Phelan J, Kellogg R. *The Nature of Narrative.* Oxford: Oxford University Press; 2006 (40th anniversary edition).
- Van Maanen J. *Tales of the Field: on writing ethnography.* Chicago, IL: University of Chicago Press; 1988.
- Weick K. *Sensemaking in Organizations.* London: SAGE Publications; 1995.

# Index